Healing Nutrition

2nd Edition

LYNN KEEGAN, PhD, RN

Director, Holistic Health Consultants
Port Angeles, Washington

DELMAR
™
THOMSON LEARNING

Australia   Canada   Mexico   Singapore   Spain   United Kingdom   United States

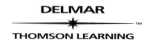

DELMAR

™

THOMSON LEARNING

Healing Nutrition, 2nd Edition
by Lynn Keegan

Health Care Publishing Director:
William Brottmiller

Product Development Manager:
Marion Waldman

Product Development Editor:
Jill Rembetski

Editorial Assistant:
Robin Irons

Executive Marketing Manager:
Dawn F. Gerrain

Channel Manager:
Gretta Oliver

Production Editor:
Mary Colleen Liburdi

Cover Design:
Mary Colleen Liburdi

Library of Congress Cataloging-in-Publication Data

ISBN: 076682571X

NOTICE TO THE READER

INTRODUCTION TO THE HEALER SERIES

LYNN KEEGAN, PhD, RN, Series Editor
Director, Holistic Health Consultants
Port Angeles, Washington

Most health care professionals care for others with compassion; they begin their formal education with this ideal. Many retain this orientation after graduation, and some manage their entire careers under this guiding principle of caring. Many of us, however, tend to forget this ideal in the hectic pace of our professional and personal lives. We may become discouraged and feel a sense of burnout.

I have spoken at many conferences with thousands of caregivers. Their experience of frustration and failure is quite common. These professionals feel themselves spread as pawns across a health care system too large to control or understand. In part, this may be because they have forgotten their true roles as healers.

When individuals redirect their personal vision and empower themselves, an entire pattern may begin to change. And so it is now with the health care profession. Most of us conceptualize our roles as much more than a vocation. We are greater than our individual roles as scientists, specialists, or care deliverers. We currently search for a name to put on our new conception of the empowered caregiver. The recently introduced term *healer* aptly describes the qualities of an increasing number of clinicians, educators, administrators, and practitioners. Today most caregivers are awakening to the realization that they have the potential for healing.

It is my feeling that, when awakened and guided to develop their own healing potential, most will function as healers. Thus, the concept of caregiver as healer is born. When we realize we have the ability to evoke others' healing, as well as care for them, a shift of consciousness begins to occur. As individual awareness and changes in skill building occur, a collective understanding of this new concept emerges. This knowledge, along with a shift in attitudes and new kinds of behavior, allows empowered health care providers to renew themselves in an expanded role. The Healer Series is born of the belief that caregivers are ready to embrace guidance that inspires them in their journeys of empowerment. Each book in the series may stand alone or be used in complementary fashion with other books. I hope and believe that information herein will strengthen you both personally and professionally, and provide you with the help and confidence to embark upon the path of a healer.

Titles in the Healer Series:

Healing Touch: A Resource for Health Care Professionals, 2nd Edition
Healing Life's Crises: A Guide for Nurses
The Nurse's Meditative Journal
Healing Nutrition
Healing the Dying, 2nd Edition
Awareness in Healing
Creative Imagery
Profiles of Nurse Healers
Healing Addictions
Healing & the Grief Process
Healing with Complementary & Alternative Therapies
Spirituality: Living Our Connectedness
Healing Meditation
Energetic Approaches to Emotional Health
Taking Charge of the Change: A Holistic Approach to the Three Phases of Menopause

To my inspiring, longtime friend
Barbara Dossey, RN, MS, FAAN,
a dynamic, nutritionally balanced, physically fit,
living example of body-mind-spirit integration.

CONTENTS

PART IV   GAINING CONTROL OF YOUR WEIGHT

PREFACE

It has been said that educators teach what they want to learn and authors write what they want to know. In the case of this book, I have been twice blessed with the opportunity to learn much about the fascinating subject of nutrition. When writing the first edition, I researched and became knowledgeable about calories, fat, vitamins, and mineral content of foods and how they affect the human body. I spent a year with the subject the first time around, and as I did so, began to understand why there are so many diseases related to nutrition. As I increased my knowledge I came to believe the reason most Americans were practically illiterate about their nutrition needs was that there was little media attention given to the topic. In the mid-1990s when I wrote the first edition, I thought that I had covered nutrition thoroughly and that this book addressed the subject in a new and interesting way. It was my hope that this book would help people know more about how nutrition can be a healing force in life—that it would make a difference.

Apparently the book did make a difference and because so many people read it and hungered for more information, the publisher and editors at Delmar Thomson asked me to write a second edition, once again pushing me to research and explore recent advances in nutrition. I hope that you will be as amazed as I am to read and discover the many advances that have only recently occurred. I was not surprised to find that many of the basic facts have remained the same so that much of the basic material can now be considered classic or perennial wisdom.

The two parts of this book that have dramatically evolved are the New Dimensions of Healing Foods and Gaining Control of Your Weight. As you read you will discover many new dimensions and documentation with cutting edge research. A detailed analysis of fad diets and their effect on health has been added to the dieting chapter. New text and research has been added to guide you in discovering resources and thus enhancing your ability to explore this fascinating subject as thoroughly as possible.

I reiterate what I stated in the first edition. As physical organisms, we are composed of millions of biochemicals. The daily input in the form of nutrients is critical to the optimal functioning of our marvelous bodies. With the newfound attention given to the topic of nutrition in the 21st century, each of us has the opportunity to become increasingly aware of information not only to prevent disease but to maximize a vital, productive life. Armed with nutrition knowledge, each of us can serve as a resource person to others. As a collective whole we can meet the objective of increased health and vitality for all people.

My hope is that the numerous books, articles, and references I have devoured to expand my understanding of this subject have become an amalgam of practical wisdom to assist you, the reader, in expanding your breadth and depth of useful information on the subject of healing nutrition. It is my additional desire that this material will be of value for both you and your clients.

—Lynn Keegan

ACKNOWLEDGMENTS

Fortunately there are always people who are present at the right place and at the right time to aid and abet us on our path through life. When I worked on the first edition of this book I had the good fortune to have a devoted editor who continually encouraged me to write, and thus together we created the best-selling first edition. When it was time to revise the content for the second edition, there was a whole new editorial team and work style in place at Delmar Thomson. The company now uses the team concept, and thus I worked closely with three people. Marion Waldman, Project Development Manager, Jill Rembetski, Project Development Editor, and Robin Irons, Editorial Assistant, were all invaluable in working with me to move this book to completion. I want to express my thanks to all three of these individuals for their ongoing help throughout the project. Publisher Bill Brottmiller continues to effectively captain a very forward-thinking crew.

Four people were chosen as reviewers for the second edition. Their insights and comments were very important to me, and I thank them for their expertise and time to review the various drafts. These reviewers are:

Cheryl Graff, MSN, RN
Nursing Instructor
Highland Community College
Baileyville, Illinois

Karilee Halo Shames, PhD, RN, HNC
Assistant Professor
Florida Atlantic University College of Nursing
Boca Raton, Florida

Dr. Marylou Martz, RN, BSN, MEd
Pennsylvania State University
Harrisburg, Pennsylvania

Barbara Merhley, MSN, PhD, RN
Nursing Instructor
Highland Community College
Freeport, Illinois

Ruth Roth, MS, RD
Associate Faculty, Indiana Purdue Fort Wayne
Clinical Dietician, Parkview Hospital
Fort Wayne, Indiana

Finally I wish to thank the numerous scientists, researchers, journalists and other media producers for their innumerable contributions in helping to awaken and evolve the field of nutrition. Because of these people, nutrition has moved from an underappreciated, little-understood subtopic to a major focus in human life in a very short period of time. At last, here in the early 2000s, almost everyone's attention is on what we individually and collectively eat and how that intake affects each of our lives and our society.

ABOUT THE AUTHOR

Many of you may have heard me speak or may have read my work in previous journal articles or books, as I have spoken at many conferences and published widely for more than 20 years. My best-known solo and coauthored book titles include:

Healing with Complementary and Alternative Therapies,
Delmar Thomson, 2001

Holistic Nursing: A Handbook for Practice, 3rd edition,
Aspen Publishers, 2000

Healing Waters: The Miraculous Health Benefits of Earth's Most Essential Resource, Berkley/Putnam Publishers, 1998

Profiles of Nurse Healers, Delmar Thomson, 1997

The Art of Caring, Sounds True, 1997

The Nurse as Healer, Delmar Thomson, 1994

I earned my bachelor's degree from Cornell University in New York, my master of science from Loma Linda University in California, and a PhD from the University of Texas at Austin. I have taught nursing at all levels at several universities and colleges, including Temple University in Philadelphia, Medical University of South Carolina, Texas Women's University, McLennan Community College in Texas, and the University of Texas Health Science Center in San Antonio. Between teaching jobs I held clinical positions, thus enabling me to continually blend theory, research, and practice.

In 1997 I was inducted as a Fellow into the American Academy of Nursing (FAAN) and in 1998 became certified as a holistic nurse (HNC). Currently, I work as an author and consultant in holistic health.

INTRODUCTION

Nutrition is our most fundamental need. We all require food and drink for basic maintenance and growth. You have probably heard the adage, "You are what you eat." Not only are we what we eat, we are also influenced by how we eat, with whom we eat, when we eat, where we eat, and why we eat. As bio-psycho-social-spiritual beings continually interacting with our environment, we are influenced by, as well as exert an influence on, our world.

Everything we do has meaning. Understanding the meaning of our daily habits, rituals, and behaviors comprises the nature of our conscious and unconscious philosophical striving. Seeking to understand nutrition and our attitudes about food is of utmost interest and concern in today's society. Why, where, when, and how we eat rank as some of our most primal questions. This book seeks to answer some of the questions about why nutrition is important and how best to provide ourselves with the optimal food for a healthy, healing life.

This book is *not* about nutritional therapy for hospitalized patients or for clients in severely compromised clinical conditions. It does not address total parenteral nutrition, enteral nutrition, or subjects such as nutritional support of the ventilator-dependent patient. This book does not contain material on diabetic exchange diets or ethical issues regarding withholding or withdrawing nutritional support. Rather, this is a book about healing nutrition to optimize a robust life.

The content is geared to maximize learning about the whys and wherefores of obtaining and eating high-quality, life-giving foods. It is designed to offer ideas to reinvigorate both the health care provider and the client. You should read this book when you are not ill, nor necessarily well, but rather in the ho-hum state of living in which so many countless millions of us spend our days. Most of us do not lack zest for living because we are nutritionally deprived, but rather because we have not optimized our potential in many realms of life, including the realm of nutrition. This book will aid you in discovering why you should pay more attention to healing nutrition, including issues such as what you are eating, where to find different food products, and the influences of why, when, where, how, and with whom you are eating.

In this book, you will find both facts and ideas. As health care professionals, we need to understand domains based on scientific models. Consequently, within this text, you will find tables and figures on which to build your knowledge base. On the other hand, much of our motivation and impetus for change comes from another dimension, a dimension emanating from the subconscious and/or super-conscious. Based on this truism, understanding healing nutrition from the paradigm of holism is also emphasized within the text. Lastly, the theme of healing is the backbone of this work. Therefore, all the content is directed toward gleaning information for self-healing and assisting others in their healing processes.

PART
I

The Importance of Healing Nutrition

Why Healing Nutrition?

HOLISM

We are holistic beings. As such, we live on multiple interacting planes. Nutrition plays an active role in each of our component parts. For example, one who eats wholesome, living, broad-spectrum foods is more likely to have a healthy physical body. One who has a healthy physical body is more likely to develop or possess a healthy spirit, mind, and emotions. Consider Figure 1–1, which depicts a holistic template that demonstrates the interrelationship of each of our holistic component parts.

Each of our daily actions affects our total health. Because of the holistic aspect of our being, each system has a direct or indirect effect on every other system. We are not static physical forms but human beings who live in continual flow and change and are constantly renewing ourselves in all areas. As we evolve, it is not only our bodies that change. We are so connected that changing the body simultaneously affects the mind and spirit. For example, when we begin to shed unwanted pounds and tighten muscle groups, we feel simultaneous lifts in our spirits and mental outlooks. On the other hand, when we accumulate more and more weight and nothing fits, we feel accompanying drops in zest and sluggishness of our spirits. Once we become aware of these concepts we begin to realize healing in any one area of being is related to all aspects of the self.

The Body-Mind-Spirit Template

As you read through this book consider all aspects of yourself. Reflect on your body, mind, and spirit and how these parts interrelate. Consider that when you feel physically ill—achy, nauseated, or feverish, for example—any one of those or other physical symptoms will impact other areas of your body. If you feel achy, most likely you are reluctant to move around. When nauseated, the inclination is to be very still. When feverish you want to decrease the temperature, so you may place a cool cloth on your face. In each of these instances, the body symptom has a direct effect on other parts of the body.

Likewise, effects of the body are felt in the mind. For example, aches and pains are likely to redirect the focus of the mind from mental tasks to how to comfort the body. There are spiritual aspects involved as well. Focus on bodily needs redirects attention that might be given to prayer or meditation. Conversely, sometimes bodily needs cause an increased emphasis on one's spiritual dimension and thus awaken and/or activate the spiritual body. Figure 1–1 is a linear example of this model. Looking at the model from another perspective, when we have a mental problem, we may neglect the body, perhaps by not paying attention to what or how we eat. Mental disturbance not only affects the mind, but also the body and spirit.

Placing spirit at the head of the list sometimes produces interesting results. For example, a person who feels spiritually elevated may take exceptionally good care of the body that carries its soul and feed nourishing mental food to the mind. Conversely, in times of spiritual ennui, the lagging spirit is reflected in a shoddy body and a disrupted mental thought process. Thus all parts of our being, body, mind, and spirit are interwoven and interrelated.

	BODY	MIND	SPIRIT
BODY	body body	mind body	spirit body
MIND	body mind	mind mind	spirit mind
SPIRIT	body spirit	mind spirit	spirit spirit

Figure 1–1 Body-mind-spirit template.
Copyright Keegan, L., & Dossey, B., 1987. Used with permission.

CASE STUDY: Nadia's Story

In 1976 Nadia Comaneci was the first woman in Olympic gymnastic history to score a perfect 10. She won one bronze medal and three gold medals. In 1979 she came to the United States to compete in the World Gymnastics Championships. Everyone expected a brilliant performance, but after a few competitive rounds, she was hospitalized with what was called a minor infection on her hand. Due to a delayed healing response, she had to remain hospitalized. Newspaper reports from the Fort Worth *Star Telegram* (December 10, 1979) revealed that Nadia had been dieting, eating only one full meal every 2 days and snacking on occasional fruits and vegetables to maintain her slim, lithe figure.

It had taken tremendous teamwork to get Nadia into this world-class position; yet the team had neglected the need for optimum nutrition. Although the team included someone who was responsible for nutrition, the gymnastic coaches were concerned with maintaining Nadia's body weight and continuing her long practice hours. As a result of the imbalance, Nadia's body became so depleted that it was unable to fight off a simple infection. The malnourished body is susceptible to infections because the immune defense system and the antibody response are decreased.

In Nadia's case, the functional breakdown came first in her body. It was only after she became ill that her coaches realized what inadequate nutrition had caused. Lack of sufficient calories affected other body functions resulting in a diminished ability to heal wounds. Only when hospitalized and despirited and depressed because she could not compete did Nadia and her caregivers understand how all parts function together and that to neglect one is to neglect the others.

A NEW RESPECT FOR FOOD

Our growing respect for the innate powers of food is actually not new; it is simply reemerging. Pharmacopoeias of ancient Egypt, Babylonia, Greece, and China were based on food. It was Hippocrates who proclaimed, "Let your food be your medicine and let your medicine be your food." Twelfth-century Jewish physician and philosopher Maimonides recommended chicken soup as a remedy for asthma. Garlic, mustard seed, and other herbs and spices collected in gardens or from the countryside were used medicinally by healers for centuries.

It was not until the modern pharmaceutical industry arose in the 19th century that we placed the obvious behind us and became enamored of manufactured stopgaps. Now as health costs have skyrocketed and the harmful side effects of drugs are becoming increasingly apparent, there is a resurgence of interest in dietary moderation and treatment with natural foods and herbs. For example, many of us might take an antacid if we have discomfort from overeating. Before this pharmacological era, we would not have had the medicine to mask this sort of symptom. We would probably have been more careful the next time not to overindulge and suffer from its untoward effects. With each passing year, there seems to be increasing awareness of the benefits of moderation and the considered use of food to prevent illness as well as to heal maladies.

THE CIRCLE OF HUMAN POTENTIAL

The dance of life involves many possibilities. I like to envision people as beings of wholeness and as such I am attracted to the model of the Circle of Human Potentials (Figure 1–2). This model comprises six areas: physical, mental, emotional, spiritual, relationships, and choices. A circle is an ancient symbol of wholeness. The circle in this model has six separate but equally important parts.

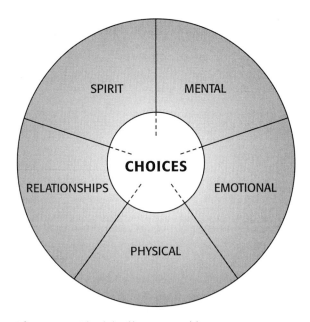

Figure 1–2 The circle of human potentials.
Copyright Keegan, L., & Dossey, B., 1987. Used with permission.

When any part is incomplete, the entire circle loses its completeness because all parts create the whole.

All of our human potentials constantly interact. When we treat our physical bodies with respect by feeding them properly and care for them by ingesting only healthy foods, we begin to change other aspects of our beings. As we become stronger by eating nutritiously, exercising, stretching, and making other physical improvements, we begin to become healthier and happier. This then impacts our other potentials.

We can learn through conscious effort how to enhance health and decrease the symptoms of disease. The idea of consciousness must be central in the continued development and understanding of our human potential. When we think of wholeness, we not only affect our attitudes toward others, but also affect our understanding of our connectedness of body, mind, and spirit.

SUMMARY

We are holistic beings, and as such we live and function on multiple interacting planes. The most commonly used terms for these planes are *body, mind,* and *spirit.* Put in a broader perspective, we can imagine all of our possibilities as a circle of human potential. Each of these dimensions, or potentials, works in harmony with the whole. Any part that is off balance, ill, or otherwise impaired influences the rest of our being.

The importance of nutrition in keeping the body in good repair is not new; what is new is the affirmation that incidences of chronic diseases have dietary links and that a good diet can help prevent as well as treat disease. Although some of us may need to enhance our food intake with supplements due to biochemical individuality, no supplement can take the place of a basic, well-rounded diet. Hippocrates was right—food is the best medicine.

CHAPTER 2

The Meaning of Food

"Hey Mom. What's for dinner?"

"I'm starving. Honey, let's go out tonight."

"It's my birthday and I want to eat the whole carton of ice cream."

"I'm taking 5 pounds off and that's all there is to it! So, no, I will not join you for lunch."

OVERVIEW

For each of us, food carries meaning. The meaning may vary from year to year, season to season, or event to event, but food is always coupled with meaning. Historically, homemakers have brought families together around tables at dinnertime. In many homes, special weekly meals are still planned following Sunday or Sabbath religious services, and celebratory meals follow major life events such as baptisms, weddings, and even funerals. Any way we look at it, food is used to commemorate significant life events. However, not all of the associations are positive. Consider, for example, the last time you were angry or sick. Do you recall a lack of appetite? Remember times of sadness or depression. These events are often coupled with anorexia, or lack of appetite. However, some of us experience the opposite reaction during times of grief and eat more than is normal. Suffice it to say that food is directly associated with both positive and negative emotions and the events linked to those emotional times. The meaning of food is inexorably intertwined with our bodies, minds, and spirits.

CHOICES

The joy of healthy nutrition is that we are part of it. We get to choose what enters our bodies. But before we can hope to select a diet intelligently, we must first learn about the values of foods, what minerals and vitamins they contain, and how our bodies use minerals and vitamins to give us great health and long lives. Every time we go to the store or sit down to a meal, we make a choice about what to eat. We learn to base these choices on what our bodies need as well as on our feelings, desires, and conditioned responses. The more information we have, the greater our ability to understand the meaning we attach to food and to make healthy choices about it.

Foods have power. Foods transfer their power to us when we digest and assimilate them. One of the basic premises underlying the ability of food to heal is that food is comprised of organic chemicals just as we are. The body's chemical structure is strikingly similar to that of seawater. However, the chemical elements in our bodies are structured in a more highly evolved order.

Unlike medicines, food enables us to build up or tear down the tissues of our bodies. When we eat well, we build strong, healthy bodies, but when our diets are defective, we tear down our bodies by destroying vital tissues. There is a power within each of us that can work miracles if we provide our bodies with the minerals and vitamins they need.

It has been known for a long time that no cell lasts longer than 7 years. What few of us know is that the majority of cells do not live nearly that long. For example, we grow several fingernails in a year; dermal skin cells take only 2 years to be replaced. Furthermore, physiologic chemists say our bodies do not contain a blood cell that is more than 14 days old. Even more amazing is that we rebuild a new heart every 30 days. That means we have a new start in life every month, a new beginning in which to provide the proper nutrition that can revitalize our bodies and our lives. By eating properly we can possibly add 10, 20, 30, or even 40 years to our life spans. Each day brings a new opportunity for a fresh start.

Our organs are destined to self-repair, but they need opportunities to do so. They will do the best they can with what we give them, even junk food. When we properly balance our diets, however, our bodies begin to respond. When taken into the body, every bit of food does one of three things:

1. It goes into building and repairing bones and tissue.
2. It supplies energy for gland secretion and for cleansing.
3. It merely passes through the digestive and elimination organs.

The number of calories we ingest are empty unless the calories come from a proper balance of food. Without a continuing variety of nutrient-enriched foods, good health cannot be achieved.

ATTITUDE

What we want to strive for, along with healthy nutrition and balanced lifestyles, are positive mental attitudes. We are all born with the potential to live long, healthy, and happy lives, but we usually fall short because of two main reasons: (1) misinformation and (2) inconsistency. Most of us simply do not adhere to lifelong regimens of wholesome diets and regular exercise. All of us need moderate regular exercise along with good diets. The point is to be consistent. It is not what we eat or drink or how we move occasionally that determines our levels of health. It is what we practice daily that determines how long and how well we will live.

We would all improve our lives tremendously if we applied what many corporations are ingraining in the minds of their employees: quality, consistency, and performance. We, as individuals, need to be conscious about the quality of our lives, know what it is that we want, have a plan for obtaining it, and have the energy to do so.

A life filled with quality work, positive thoughts, loving friends, and activity tends to strengthen our natural immunity to germs, viruses, and negative hereditary influences. A positive attitude works hand in hand with good nutrition. Healing nutrition can work, rebuilding our bodies from the inside out as we open them to the interrelationship of mental, spiritual, and emotional aspects of food's curative powers. The effectiveness of healing food has been clinically proven by research and thousands of individual case histories. The way to begin is to feel a true harmony with life in our hearts, a harmony set free by the knowledge about what will bring quality into our lives every hour of every day that we spend on this earth.

Every acute disease episode is a healing crisis. It results when the body struggles to free itself of toxins. Nature does her best to keep the body clean, but we must help. Every insect and animal has a natural instinct for self-preservation. The farther up the animal chain, the more this instinct is lost. Ironically, as animals, our instincts are often safer than our intelligence. When an animal is sick it eats nothing, or it eats only grass. In effect, it purges its body of toxins. Many foods do produce remarkable short-term benefits. However, it is only with consistent proper nutrition and exercise of the body, along with the proper state of mind, that we can achieve a state of wellness that safeguards against imbalance in our systems and contributes to disease prevention. It is certainly possible that healing foods that can prevent an illness can also cure an illness.

QUALITY OF LIFE

Ask yourself: On the whole, am I as healthy as I can be? Are those with whom I live and work healthy? Before you answer, visualize the last time you were in a committee meeting or at a large conference. In your mind's eye, look at the people.

Were they physically fit? Did they look tired and haggard? What did their skin look like? Were their eyes clear and bright? And what about the older people? Were they energetic and full of life or worn out and tired of living? Now, how about you? Are you filled with zest and vitality, or is there room for improvement? Is your quality of life what you want it to be? The easiest place to begin is with your physical body, with what you put into your mouth. Most of us want quality of life. Through a change in dietary habits, we can achieve it. The remarkable by-product is that, with effort, not only do we improve the quality of our lives, but we are also likely to increase our satisfaction with our lives.

HUMAN EVOLUTION

Humans evolved over millions of years, and this evolution was shaped by many factors, including climate, habitat, and the ability to adapt to the environment. Early people were hunter-gatherers, living off fruits, nuts, and plants and hunting animals for food and clothing. Their food was rich in nutrients and loaded with the necessary life-giving energy. The fact is that the human species has remained relatively unchanged for the last 40,000 years. Our physiological makeup is the same as that of our Stone Age ancestors. For the most part, Stone Age people were lean, strong, aerobically fit, and almost totally free of the chronic diseases that cause 75 percent of all deaths in the United States today. Changes in human nutrition and exercise patterns have contributed to cancer, heart disease, diabetes, hypertension, obesity, and even the tooth decay that we have today. In the Stone Age, death was seldom caused by degenerative disease because the average life span of Stone Age people was shorter than that of contemporary people. Instead, death likely came from confrontations with animals, life-threatening injuries, or natural disasters.

Forty thousand years ago, people lived in seminomadic tribes. They moved with the seasons, following game, water, and plant foods. They were lean and strong and dependent on their stamina and strength for survival. Although their diet was occasionally insufficient in quantity, they usually had enough to eat, and most importantly their food was rich in life-giving nutrients. Those who survived the assault of accidents and infections could look forward to a long and fit life, untroubled by the degenerative diseases that afflict modern humans. The point is that our Stone Age ancestors did not die of the same diseases that recently have caused most of the deaths in the United States, and yet, physiologically, they were identical to us. The primary differences between them and us, other than some environmental factors, are the activity levels and foods we eat. Through various processes over the last 40,000 years, our food supply has changed. The way our ancestors lived was relatively the same for over a million years, but then something happened. This event was not the Ice Age or a meteor striking the planet. No, this event was far more significant because what happened biologically changed the Earth and altered the destiny of humankind forever.

About 10,000 years ago, some of our ancestors abandoned their age-old hunting and gathering way of life for a more settled existence based on agriculture and, eventually, on animal husbandry. Humans began to grow their own food. Like a genie let out of a bottle, powerful and unprecedented forces were unleashed: forces unlike those that had controlled the ecology and evolution of plants, animals, and microorganisms during the preceding 3 billion years. This event, known as the Neolithic Revolution, transformed our planet.

Once introduced, agriculture prevailed as the leading mode of human subsistence and was a very efficient way of feeding larger groups of people. With agriculture, humans began to flourish, and as a people, we began to control our food supply. We had more time to develop our cultures. Civilizations were created. Science, art, and the quest for enlightenment expanded. The planet was transformed. Today we are the beneficiaries of these changes.

As humans discovered agriculture and began cooking, processing, and storing food, modern health problems slowly began to surface. Diseases that never existed began to afflict human beings. We had better shelter, warmer clothing, and, most important, plenty of food. Where were these new diseases coming from? Remember, for millions of years humans evolved by eating only what they could gather, forage, or kill. The relationship with food was based solely on survival. Think about that for a moment. Before agriculture was introduced, humans ate only to survive. Our bodies' evolution was the result of food that was present in the natural world. In that natural world, life existed based only on what it needed to survive. Now, with the sudden abundance of food, that perfect relationship that exists only in nature was changed as people began to eat for pleasure. They ate because they wanted to eat. When the desire to eat changed from need to want, the natural state of human health was never the same again.

As people became more skilled at raising crops and domesticating animals, foods became plentiful, and the variety of choices increased as well. These choices were based on a new variable: taste. Then, inevitably, came the intentional manipulation and creation of foods based on markets for things that tasted good. Remember, for millions of years, humans ate foods that were available from hunting or foraging, foods that were rich in nutrients to which the human body had carefully adapted, foods that the body was programmed to digest with the help of nature. Selection and choice were limited and driven by hunger; the purpose of eating was to survive.

Think of this connection between taste, evolution, and the manipulation of our food supply. The taste of food is merely a biological mechanism that tells the brain what foods to eat and what foods not to eat. In general, foods that had energy and nutrients to sustain life were foods that tasted good. Nuts and berries that were too sour or too bitter were poisonous, or at least unripe, and were therefore not good nutrient choices. These foods were discarded because they were not pleasant to eat. By using the sense of taste, humans unconsciously selected the proper foods that would nourish them and discarded substances that would not nourish them. The power of our sense of taste is truly amazing.

In the natural world, survival is the first priority. Every function of every living organism has one primary overriding objective—survival. Taste is one of the survival mechanisms developed over millions of years to help us select nutrient-rich foods and to eat them in sufficient quantities to ensure survival. So, what does it all mean? What do taste buds and cavepeople have to do with living to a healthful old age? The answer is "everything." Taste drives us to pick certain foods. Evolution formed a powerful connection between our taste buds and our brains, and this happened not in the last 100 years but over millions of years. When we eat something that tastes good, our bodies signal our brains that this food is necessary for survival and our brains tell us yes, that is good, eat more, eat as much as we can, because in the natural world, our next meal may be a long way off. That was then, however, and this is now.

The difference today is that foods that taste good are not always good for us. As we humans became skilled at growing food and domesticating animals, we literally altered the natural world. Foods were genetically altered in large part to satisfy our sense of taste. We learned the art of hybridization to a degree that many of the foods we used to eat as a species no longer exist today. Grains such as corn and wheat, as well as the livestock we eat today, are not the same as those of 1,000 years ago or even 100 years ago.

The objective of the modern food manufacturing business, like any industry, is to create products that will satisfy markets and create profits. To meet these objectives, the food industry has created foods that taste good so that we will buy them. On the surface, this may seem relatively harmless. If you think about it, the result of millions of years of evolution, in which there was this perfect relationship between humans and their food supply, suddenly changed. The slightly salty taste of a natural root or nut, the semisweet flavor of a wild berry, or the warm and succulent taste of wild game all send signals to our brains, triggering a desire to eat. This perfectly natural biological mechanism that was designed to ensure survival is now being used to select foods with exaggerated flavors. What is amazing is that we are talking about three basic tastes: the tastes of fat, sugar, and salt. Think about it. A thick, juicy steak, heavy butter and cream sauces, and rich desserts all contain excessive amounts of fat, sugar, and salt, foods that did not even exist a thousand years ago. Why do humans crave these kinds of foods, and why do we become obsessed with eating them?

To better understand, let us look at each taste in terms of human nutrition. Fats, sugar, and salt comprise the tastes that guide most of our food choices.

Fat

Fats are a necessary part of our diets. They contain essential fatty acids that are needed to formulate hundreds of chemicals in our bodies. They also make up the components of our entire hormone system. Fats are needed to prevent inflammation, lubricate joints, and form the linings of cells. Certain fats help remove cholesterol from arteries, transport certain vitamins to hungry cells, and help the immune systems fight disease. Fat is also used as stored energy. When fat is not used at the time of consumption, it is stored by our bodies in special fat cells. When food is not readily available for an extended period of time, and the body needs energy, fat is converted into fuel. This method of energy storage evolved over millions of years of human history and was vital to survival during lean periods when food sources were scarce.

In the ancient natural world, fat was very hard to come by. Seeds, nuts, plants, fish, and wild game were the only fat sources available. This factor, combined with an inconsistent and occasionally scarce food supply, forced nature to develop a strong connection between our sense of taste and our desire to eat foods that are good sources of fat. When humans began selecting foods based on taste, foods high in fat became the foods of choice. Think about the fatty foods available to us now, like fat-laden red meat from domesticated cattle or butter and cream from dairy cows. Those foods did not exist a thousand years ago and do not occur naturally in nature.

Sugar

Sugar is divided into two categories: complex carbohydrates and simple carbohydrates. Complex carbohydrates such as vegetables, fruits, and grains occur naturally. An example of a simple carbohydrate is white refined sugar. It is processed from sugarcane, and has no nutritional value other than to supply calories. Natural complex carbohydrates are the best sources of energy. Unlike simple carbohydrates, they metabolize slowly, providing a steady flow of fuel to keep us alert. Nature knew that. When we found this amazing energy fuel, we needed to eat it. Again, a strong connection between our sense of taste and a desire to eat carbohydrates developed.

Salt

Salt, the third major taste, is also crucial to our bodies. It maintains the balance of our body fluids, preventing dehydration by regulating key hormones. It helps the heart, the kidneys, and the adrenal glands to monitor all of our bodily functions. Salt helps maintain blood pressure and is necessary to the body's electrical system.

Salt occurs naturally in most foods, and it is those natural salts that our bodies crave and need. It is important to note that the organic salts found in plants and animals are not the same as table salt. The connection between taste and the desire to eat substances containing salt was established long ago in our brains. When preagricultural humans found organic substances that contained fat, sugar, and salt, their brains told them to eat and to eat a lot of the substances.

Through the process of evolution, survival of the human species depended on foods that possessed one or all of the three characteristics of taste. When we gained control of our food supply, we began to alter foods to satisfy our tastes. The foods we routinely choose to eat contain significantly more fat, sugar, and salt than occur naturally. Because our sense of taste and hunger connection is so strong, the concentration of fat, sugar, and salt in those foods increases dramatically.

What does all this mean? It simply means this: Powerful biological mechanisms drive us to seek foods that are rich in fat, salt, and sugar and in our modern world, the foods that contain these substances are not what nature intended us to eat. These foods trick our bodies into believing they are receiving nutrition when most of the foods contain useless empty calories. As a result, it is this concentration of fat, sugar, and salt in the foods we eat that contributes to the increased occurrences of heart disease, cancer, hypertension, stroke, diabetes, kidney failure, and osteoporosis. Concerns about nutrition and health have expanded within recent years beyond the need to prevent deficiencies. In other words, our typical U.S. diet is not only providing us with improper nutrition, it is killing us, slowly and insidiously.

The nutritionally related diseases of coronary heart disease, stroke, cancer, and diabetes are the leading causes of death and disability in the United States. Substantial scientific research over the past few decades indicates that diet can play an important role in preventing such conditions. Remember the expression, "You are what you eat." The only source of raw material for the cells in our bodies to replicate and continue life is contained in the foods we eat. Whether we realize it or not, what we put into our bodies in large measure determines the length and the quality of our lives.

Understanding this, we may surmise that our very lives depend on what we eat. A diet high in fat can clog our arteries and restrict the flow of blood to and from our hearts. Eventually our hearts are overworked and our cells do not receive the nutrition they need to function properly and renew themselves. We may then become one of the millions of people who suffer from coronary heart disease. Likewise, a diet high in refined sugar can lead to diabetes, obesity, kidney failure, depression, and cancer. For many people, too much salt can be deadly. Salt causes the body to retain excess water, and because the body can only hold a limited amount of fluid, the heart is strained tremendously. Excess salt can lead to kidney damage as well as a host of other complications.

LIFE EXTENSION

The search for the fountain of youth is as old as humankind. From ancient culture to modern civilization, extending the human life span has changed from an elusive dream to a present-day reality. The secret of maximizing life expectancy and living youthfully well into old age, the 90s and beyond, is not found in a synthesized new drug or bionic body part; the key is the foods we eat.

I was first exposed to the idea of life expansion through the theories of Durk Pearson and Sandy Shaw (1982) described in their book *Life Extension*. My initial reaction was that their method seemed risky: too many supplements and too little scientific validation. The idea of life extension repopularized in the 20th century by Pearson and Shaw generated many more books and abundant research. Examples of best-selling books that followed *Life Extension* include *Longevity: The Science of Staying Young* (Keeton, 1992) and Gary Null's *Ultimate Anti-Aging Program* (1999).

To many, old age brings senility, incontinence, and chronic illness often with concomitant pain and misery until death finally occurs. Who wants to live like that? Chronological age may not, in fact, have to be linked with cellular age. Cellular age can be defined as the age of the cells in our bodies. What if being 80 meant looking and feeling as if you were a 40-year-old who has the vitality of a 20- or 30-year-old? Imagine living well past 100 without any illness or disease because your cells function as if they were decades younger. Think about having multiple careers and pursuing new hobbies or enjoying romantic interests well into your 90s and beyond. Consider what that could mean. How many people work hard all of their lives and never get to enjoy the money and leisure for which they labored? Imagine being young and vital at 65 and living a full and healthful life.

One of the goals of this book is to help you learn how to healthfully live out your maximum life span. This means not just adding years but stretching out the periods of youth and middle age so that at 80 calendar years, the cells in our bodies function as those of a youthful 40-year-old, full of energy and vitality. Whatever our reasons may be for wanting to live younger longer, it may actually be possible to reverse the symptoms of aging and extend our life spans by doing one very simple thing: Make the decision to consistently adjust our eating habits.

Food is the giver of life. Sickness does occur because of genetics, germs, or just plain bad luck, but the vast majority of all illness is the result of how we choose to live our lives. The results of the choices we make regarding the food we eat, which to a large extent we have more control over than any other factor, determine how long we will live and the quality of life we will have. Until you have experienced it, you may understand this principle on an intellectual level but not necessarily on the deeper emotional level. In other words, until we feel more alive and healthier than we have ever felt, these are just words that have little meaning. The secret to living younger longer is not about transplanted organs, surgery, or synthetic drugs; it is about strengthening the physiology within our bodies. Life extension is about erasing the errors of years of eating lifeless, highly processed foods and feeding our bodies the vital nutrients they need on a cellular level to increase vital functions and ward off infection and disease.

Models for Life Extension

Nothing definite has been demonstrated to slow or reverse the primary aging process in humans; instead, the factors that are known to affect longevity do so by their influence on disease development, which is part of secondary aging. Preventive strategies against secondary aging are aimed at maintaining health and functional capacity, rather than extending the survival curve. To date, interventions for preventive geriatrics and successful aging include a low-fat diet with a high content of fruits and vegetables; exercise; and hormone replacement (Holloszy, 2000). However, new models are currently under investigation.

CALORIC RESTRICTION

One of the most robust observations in the biology of aging is that caloric restriction (CR) extends life in a variety of species (Barzilai & Gupta, 1999). CR can be defined as reducing the total level of calories consumed. This reduction needs to be individually calculated based on one's age and physical activity. CR is the most successful method of extending both median and maximal life spans in rodents and other short-lived species. It is not yet clear whether this method of life extension will be successful in longer-lived species, including humans; however, trials on rhesus monkeys are underway (Pendergrass et al., 1999).

Previous studies of CR have tended to start after weaning and the effects of prenatal or early postnatal diet restriction have rarely been considered. However, existing literature suggests that reducing nutrition at this earlier stage of life has opposite effects, resulting in accelerated aging and a reduction in life span. These findings support emerging epidemiological evidence in humans that poor nutrition in early life may program accelerated aging and predispose individuals to a variety of age-related diseases (Aihie Sayer & Cooper, 1997).

Using the dietary restriction paradigm as a prototype, it is possible that a three-pathway model may provide the bases to enhance life extension: (1) retardation of biological aging, (2) suppression of age-related disease, and (3) modulation of cross talk between the first two. Another useful concept in relation to interventions is the enhancement of natural resistance in order to deter an organism's vulnerability to aging and disease. These models are best used to explain the efficacy of currently popular interventions such as antioxidant supplementation and hormone therapies. Such interventions highlight the promises that antioxidant supplements hold in warding off oxidative damage as well as their inherent problems and biological limitations. Also possible are antiaging interventions by genetic manipulation, as seen in animal model studies, and prophylactic treatments targeted against disease, such as hormonal approaches using estrogen and DHEA, as well as other intervening measures (Yu, 1999).

THE ROLE OF FAT MASS IN LIFE EXTENSION

Although CR results in a several-fold decrease in fat mass (FM), the role of fat in life extension has traditionally been considered minimal. Two main reasons accounted for this belief. First, although increased FM is associated with changes in substrate oxidation and in glucose homeostasis, in part through the effects of free fatty acids (FFA) and glycerol, several studies have suggested that longevity is determined independent of FM. Second, CR has systemic effects on a range of functions including neurological, endocrine, reproductive, immunological, and antineoplastic, none of which have been historically linked to fat. In the last few years, an explosion of evidence has demonstrated that fat tissue is a result of a very active endocrine gland which secretes a variety of peptides (such as leptin and plasminogen activating inhibitor-1), cytokines (such as tumor necrosis factor), and complement factors. This is in addition to the presence of substrates, such as glycerol and FFA, which are stored and released by fat cells and are known to have a major role in hepatic and peripheral glucose metabolism. This research suggests that many of the systemic effects of CR can now be explained by the chronic effects related to decreased plasma levels of peptides, cytokines, complement factors, and substrates. In fact, all of the benefits of CR on the neuroendocrine system and those related to the improvement in glucose homeostasis can be attributed to decrease in adipose cells and their products. Other evidence from epidemiological data in human obesity supports the role of FM and its body distribution as a risk factor for morbidity and mortality in humans due to impaired glucose metabolism (similar to rodents), for cancer (similar to rodents), and for the development of atherosclerotic vascular disease (in humans). If all or most of the life-extending benefits of CR can be attributed to decreased fat stores, the expression of specific candidate proteins may be explored and manipulated in the search for the most powerful adipose-dependent signals that modulate life expectancy (Barzilai & Gupta, 1999).

CONSCIOUS DECISIONS

The key to a program of healing nutrition is making conscious efforts to eliminate or reduce foods that harm our bodies. No matter how hard we try to defend today's food choices, we must realize that most of these foods did not even exist 100 years ago. The truth is that our bodies are not really designed to eat these foods in the quantities that we do. The taste and hunger for fat, sugar, and salt in the Stone Age meant searching for food choices that would ensure survival. In the modern world, those same tastes and hungers led us to develop processed foods that are almost totally devoid of nutritional value but that taste good. Today we eat tons of great-tasting, lifeless food. Most of us never make the connection between the food we eat and how we feel physically until it is too late.

In 1754 philosopher Jean-Jacques Rousseau wrote that in a state of nature, men were strong of limb, fleet of foot, and clear of eye. Today, most of our ills are of our own making, and we might have avoided them by adhering to that simple manner of life prescribed by nature. The simple truth is that nature has provided us with all the basic means from which to build our bodies from birth to old age in a state of maximum health, to enjoy life experiences with abundant energy, vigor, and vitality, and to achieve a happy, long life span. The secret, which is really no secret at all, consists of making conscious decisions to put the right foods into our mouths at the right times. Only then will we have optimal nourishment and a proper state of mind. Right now, at the highest levels of government, our leaders are seeking ways to finance a system of health care that could cost a trillion dollars to treat all of the sick and dying citizens afflicted with the degenerative diseases of modern humans. Yet the cure for many of these ills is already available to us. It is not a miracle drug therapy, and it is not expensive. It is the food we eat and making the connection in our minds between the foods we eat today and the sickness and health that result years down the road.

Do no harm to your body. The meaning of that phrase seems obvious. People who care about their personal welfare would probably not intentionally harm their bodies. For example, would you stick your hand in a fire or walk into the path of oncoming traffic? These conscious acts are obviously potentially harmful to our bodies, but what about the potentially harmful things we do every day and never think about? Consider those unconscious acts we perform every time we sit down to eat. Doing no harm means we need to be consciously aware of any potential risk that could result from the kinds of foods we eat. It is not that we should never eat these foods, but that we should be conscious of what to eat daily. Strive to consciously limit those foods that contain excessive fat, sugar, and salt and to focus on foods that feed your cells super nutrition. An easy rule to remember is that before you put anything into your mouth, ask yourself one simple question—Will eating this food make my body feel good? Then make your choice about eating it based on your answer.

When we walk into any modern supermarket we are faced with over 30,000 food choices. As we wheel our carts past the meat counter, the microwave section, through the canned food section, and past the salty snack and the dairy sections, we end up in the produce aisle where most of our best food choices are located. Even the produce we choose today is not the same as that of our ancestors. It probably looks better because it has been polished and waxed. Remember that years of genetic engineering have gone into creating foods and vegetables that look good and have a long shelf life. Many of these foods are grown in mineral-deprived soils. Even though this produce looks perfect and tastes good, it is not the same as it once was 1,000 years ago.

We are faced with myriad food choices of which only a very few are really any good for us. Many are either neutral or harmful. By paying a little closer attention to foods that are potentially harmful, we may be able to add significant quality years to our lives. It is important to remember that the foods to reduce are those which contain saturated fats, added salts, refined sugars, caffeine, and chemical additives. We will discuss each of these foods in the following chapters.

SUMMARY

The foods we put into our bodies affect how we look and feel, and even impacts our potential life spans. We have so many choices about food—what, where, when, how, and with whom we eat. A winning attitude of positive thoughts and effective decision making can impact the quality of life.

Humans have long sought an elixir to long life. Through a complex human evolutionary cycle humankind has finally arrived on the threshold of genuine capacity for life extension. New models and theories for expanding human life are currently under scientific scrutiny and each year more information becomes available. With so many new alternatives emerging, health care providers will want to make conscious decisions. There are many options to add meaning and thus enhance the quality of life both for ourselves and for our clients. I invite you to continue to read about a new way of living that will increase you potential life span and help you to be healthier for the rest of your natural life.

REFERENCES

Aihie Sayer, A., & Cooper, C. (1997). Undernutrition and aging. *Gerontology, 43*(4), 203–205.

Barzilai, N., & Gupta, G. (1999). Revisiting the role of fat mass in the life extension induced by caloric restriction. *Journal of Gerontology Annals of Biological and Medical Sciences, 54*(3), B89–96; discussion B97–98.

Eat to live 120 years. (1992). Redmond, WA: Zygon International.

Harman, D. (1998). Extending functional life span. *Experimental Gerontology, 33*(1–2), 95–112.

Holloszy, J. O. (2000). The biology of aging. *Mayo Clinic Proceedings, 75,* S3–8; discussion S8–9.

Keeton, K. (1992). *Longevity: the science of staying young.* New York: Viking.

Null, G. (1999). *Ultimate anti-aging program.* New York: Kensington.

Pearson, D., & Shaw, S. (1982). *Life extension: A practical scientific approach.* New York: Warner Books.

Pendergrass, W. R., Lane, M. A., Bodkin, N. L., Hansen, B. C., Ingram, D. K., Roth, G. S., Yi, L., Bin, H., & Wolf, N. S. (1999). Cellular proliferation potential during aging and caloric restriction in rhesus monkeys (Macaca mulatta). *Journal of Cellular Physiology, 180*(1), 123–130.

U.S. Department of Health & Human Services. (1988). *The Surgeon General's report on nutrition and health.* DHHS (PHS) Publication No. 88–50211.

Willix, R. (1994). *3 minutes a day to a 120 year lifespan.* Baltimore, MD: Health for Life.

Yu, B.P. (1999). Approaches to anti-aging intervention: The promises and the uncertainties. *Mechanisms of Ageing and Development, 111*(2–3), 73–87.

Food and Disease

The goal of healing nutrition is to maximize body-mind-spirit health. If we neglect nutritional self-care and add to the situation heredity and environmental factors, certainly disease and illness may occur. I group some of these beginning, non-life-threatening ailments into the category of "benign self-neglect." These seemingly benign disorders, if left unattended, have the potential to evolve into full-blown illnesses or diseases.

Detrimental nutritional states result from both undernutrition and overconsumption. Those who overconsume not only will be overweight, they may also be undernourished.

BENIGN SELF-NEGLECT

The concept of benign self-neglect is derived not because the outcomes are benign, but rather because the person who functions with a self-care deficit usually does so from an unaware or uninformed state of consciousness. We do not indulge in poor eating habits on purpose but rather because we do not know any better, have suppressed our knowledge in lieu of seemingly more important current events, or no longer have the motivation or desire for self-care. For example, the teenager with acne may be uninformed about the deleterious effects of junk food and inadequate skin hygiene. Young parents may be so busy chauffeuring, tutoring, and financing their children's rearing that they may, due to simple psychological overload, sit and eat chips, dips, candy, and sodas during breaks without the kids. The fast track, upwardly mobile, career executive may believe that it is necessary to relax by having several drinks and a high-fat meal to unwind at the end of each busy workday. All of these individuals consciously think they are doing the best they can. The teen is concentrating on schoolwork, the parent on raising children, and the executive on fulfilling career ambitions. None of them purposely mistreat their bodies. They are simply so busy concentrating on their lives' work that they fail to pause and consider the importance of good nutrition in their lives.

COMMON DISORDERS

The category of benign self-neglect includes a host of ailments. The ones most easily recognized are dental caries, fatigue, overweight, and constipation. These and other common disorders are detailed in this section. One disorder that is not so commonly recognized but of great importance is eye health. In the next section, macular degeneration is used as an example of how nutrition and benign self-neglect due to lack of information can have serious implications. This condition is heavily documented as an example of how each of the other conditions can be researched and validated.

Acne

THE PROBLEM

Acne is a disorder of the oil glands in the skin and is characterized by the recurring formation of blackheads, whiteheads, and pimples on the face and upper trunk. The incidence is greatest in puberty and adolescence when the hormones influencing the secretion of these specific oil glands are at their peak level of activity.

INTERVENTIONS

Food choices during the teen years can affect the severity of the condition. A diet high in fat and refined sugars should be avoided. This means limiting intake of soft drinks, fried foods, desserts, and nuts. It has also been found that foods rich in oxalic acid, such as chocolate, spinach, and rhubarb, may inhibit the absorption of calcium. Because calcium is important in maintaining the acid-alkali balance of the blood, which is necessary for a clear complexion, these foods should be avoided if adolescent acne is a problem.

Vitamins A and B-complex are important to healthy, glowing skin. Both vitamins are often prescribed after the fact, so why wait? Encourage young people to eat foods high in these essential vitamins. Vitamin A clears the face while B-complex vitamins, especially riboflavin (B_2), pyridoxine (B_6), and pantothenic acid, help to reduce facial oiliness and blackhead formation.

Vitamins C, D, and E and the mineral zinc also work to keep complexions healthy. Vitamin C aids in resisting the spread of infection while vitamin D safeguards the body's store of calcium from excretion. Vitamin E prevents scarring, while zinc is an effective bacterial suppressor. To see which foods provide the vitamins and minerals discussed in this chapter, refer to Chapter 8, Tables 8–1 and 8–2 (on pages 98–100 and 104–105).

Allergies

THE PROBLEM

Many people suffer from sensitivity to allergens. Allergens arise from pollens, molds, animal dander, chemicals, insect bites, and foods. Susceptibility to allergens is related to multiple factors, including heredity, stress, infections, and nutritional status. Healthy bodies are more likely to resist allergens, while inadequately nourished ones may possess weakened immune systems with increased cell permeability. This allows easy access to cell entrance by allergenic foreign substances.

INTERVENTIONS

To combat allergies, the best method is to maintain a well-balanced healthy diet and avoid known allergens.

Body Odor

THE PROBLEM

External body odors are related to the internal health of the body.

INTERVENTIONS

Certain nutrients seem to metabolically remove body wastes that cause odors. They include vitamins B_6 and PABA and the minerals magnesium and zinc.

Bruises

THE PROBLEM

Bruises are caused by the rupture of small blood vessels, resulting in discoloration of underlying tissues without a break in the overlying skin. Individuals who bruise easily, and have seen their health care practitioners to make certain they do not have diseases such as anemia or leukemia and do not use anticoagulants (like daily aspirin), should consider dietary factors.

INTERVENTIONS

Vitamin C and the bioflavonoids strengthen the small blood vessels. Vitamin K is a natural blood-clotting agent. The antioxidants, vitamins A, C, E, B_1, B_5, and B_6, and the minerals zinc and selenium are also effective in combating the rupture of small vessels.

Bruxism (Teeth Grinding)

THE PROBLEM

The annoying condition of bruxism is one that most people think is beyond their control because it usually occurs during sleep. The unfortunate effects include enamel loss, gum recession, and awakening with a tight jaw.

INTERVENTIONS

Although bruxism may be a condition that occurs primarily due to stress, certain vitamins and minerals may help. Calcium is effective for treating involuntary movements of muscles, while pantothenic acid aids in maintaining motor coordination. Both nutrients are also antistress formulas.

Colds

THE PROBLEM

The common cold is an annoying and always inconvenient occurrence. This highly contagious condition causes a general inflammation of the mucous membranes of the respiratory passages and is caused by a variety of viruses. The difficulty in curing the common cold is related to the multiple, constantly mutating viruses that are difficult to pinpoint.

INTERVENTIONS

The best prevention of the common cold is to maintain the body at high nutritional and low stress levels and wash hands frequently. We should get adequate sleep and eat diets that invigorate the immune system. When a cold strikes, certain vitamins are thought to be helpful. Some authorities, the most notable being Linus Pauling, have considered vitamin C intake to be essential in both the prevention and treatment of colds. Prevention doses are from 1 to 2 grams daily, while as much as 600 to 625 milligrams every 3 hours (when awake) may be successful for treatment. It is important to note that the controversial reports do change with ongoing research.

Constipation

THE PROBLEM

Countless people suffer from the mostly unnecessary condition of constipation. This disorder is characterized by a decreased frequency of bowel movements resulting in waste matter remaining in the colon and becoming dry and difficult to expel.

INTERVENTIONS

This condition, like many of the others, is related to simple body-mind-spirit behaviors. Constipation results from insufficient muscle tone in the bowel and/or abdominal wall that occurs due to poor habits. Lack of exercise, repeated failure to pay attention to and follow the body's signal to eliminate, insufficient fluid intake, or a diet lacking in roughage or fiber can all contribute to this disorder.

Food and body-mind training can prevent or correct this condition. Fruits, vegetables, and whole grains contain the high fiber necessary to create the needed bulk. Unsaturated fats are useful because they effectively lubricate the mucous walls of the colon. The allicin in garlic stimulates the walls of the intestines. Yogurt, buttermilk, and other milk products containing acidophilus cultures are beneficial in maintaining proper intestinal flora, especially during antibiotic therapy. Apples, papayas, pineapples, prunes, and figs also target intestinal motility. Needless to say, six to eight glasses of water a day (not teas, coffees, and sodas) are necessary to maintain adequate hydration.

Body-mind training is essential in this condition. Learning to heed the body's signal and discipline the system for a regular morning or start-of-day elimination time is part of curing this condition. Harmonizing the body with regular exercise is also essential to reverse or prevent constipation.

Dandruff

THE PROBLEM

Dandruff may be only dry flakes that occur when brushing hair or it may be a more serious condition, seborrheic dermatitis. Simple dandruff is the result of an inadequate diet and inefficient carbohydrate metabolism.

INTERVENTIONS

Dandruff can usually be reversed with a diet of unrefined carbohydrates and B vitamins. The antioxidants, vitamins C and E, and the mineral selenium are also helpful (see Chapter 8 for more information about antioxidants). Naturally, body-mind behaviors such as recognizing the need for a specialized shampoo and frequent washing and hair brushing are essential.

Dermatitis

THE PROBLEM

Dermatitis is an inflammatory, frequently recurring skin reaction. One form of dermatitis is eczema, an eruption of blisters on the skin that weep and crust. Itching, flaking, scaling, and eventual thickening and color changes of the skin may occur. This ailment, like the others, originates in body-mind-spirit behaviors. It may be associated with hereditary allergic traits and can be aggravated by stress and fatigue.

INTERVENTIONS

If the irritant is a food item, it should be eliminated from the diet. Foods rich in the B vitamins have been found to cure infants who have dermatitis. Vitamin A is also essential for maintaining healthy skin.

Diarrhea

THE PROBLEM

Valuable vitamins and minerals can be lost through frequent, loose stools. Diarrhea can be caused by bacteria or viruses in contaminated food, emotional distress, food allergies, a diet too high in roughage, or overuse of laxatives or caffeine.

INTERVENTIONS

When diarrhea occurs, supplement with vitamins C, B-complex, and sodium, magnesium, and potassium, which are lost through dehydration. Naturally, you want to take in copious fluids to replace the water lost through the stools.

Environmental Pollution

THE PROBLEM

We are continually exposed to pollutants in the air we breathe, the water we drink, and the food we eat. It is often years before the deleterious effects of these pollutants are realized. The results of these exposures range from birth defects to yellow teeth to plubism (lead poisoning).

INTERVENTIONS

Some nutrients lessen the adverse effects of pollutants. The free radical scavengers, vitamins A, C, and E, provide some protection. Vitamin C also removes lead from bone and brain tissue, as well as prevents some of the carcinogenic nitrosamines from forming. Selenium has been found to protect against mercury poisoning.

Fatigue
THE PROBLEM

Who does not know what this means and how it feels? Unfortunately, it is all too often related to whole body health and, in large part, inadequate nutrition.

INTERVENTIONS

The fast track to putting the zip back into your life includes formulating and following a balanced food program and daily movement regime. Correct deficiencies in B-complex, C, D, or iron to combat fatigue. The minerals magnesium and potassium may be supplemented to boost the muscles' ability to contract.

Flatulence
THE PROBLEM

Lots of folks pass gas. The two most common causes are gulping air while eating and releasing of gases liberated by the putrefactive bacteria living on undigested food. Another cause is the deficiency of the enzyme lactose which assists in digesting milk products. During the aging process, enzyme production often decreases, causing flatulence to develop during the "graying" years. See Chapter 10 for more information regarding enzyme supplements for aging.

INTERVENTIONS

A diet of high-fiber foods, especially apples, cabbage, brussels sprouts, and beans, will often induce flatulence due to the fibrous food remains fermenting in the intestines.

Pantothenic acid has been shown to relieve intestinal gas while the B vitamins aid in bowel motility. Yogurt and other milk products containing acidophilus bacillus aid in the digestion of high-fiber foods and replace friendly intestinal bacteria that may have been lost during diarrhea or destroyed during antibiotic therapy. Refer also to the use of herbs in Chapter 13.

Hair Health
THE PROBLEM

Dull, thinning hair is no fun. Although heredity and age play a significant role in hair loss, hair quality is, in fact, related to nutrition.

INTERVENTIONS

Protein deficiency affects hair color, texture, and quantity. When protein intake is boosted, hair quality often improves. Vitamins A, B$_6$, biotin, and folic acid are also essential for healthy hair. Women who use birth control pills (BCP) or are in their last months of pregnancy sometimes experience hair loss. This may be attributed to an imbalance of copper. The hair regrows following delivery or when the BCPs are switched or discontinued.

Halitosis

THE PROBLEM

Bad breath can be caused by improper diet, respiratory infection, sinus infection, poor oral hygiene, alcohol intake, or smoking. In some cases, it may be related to ingested chemicals such as arsenic, lead, bismuth, or methane. Even nervous tension can be the cause, but it is usually attributed to expulsion of gas from putrefactive bacteria through the mouth.

INTERVENTIONS

In addition to proper oral hygiene, a carefully regulated diet is essential to combat this socially disastrous disorder. Vitamin C is necessary to ensure oral health and prevent scurvy, while vitamin A is needed for the overall development and robust maintenance of the gums and teeth.

Headache

THE PROBLEM

Headaches may be one of the most annoying manifestations of benign self-neglect. Headaches cause misery to millions on a daily basis. Tension headaches result from contractions of the neck, scalp, or forehead muscles; vascular headaches come from uneven dilation of cerebral vessels; and sinus headaches are caused by inflamed mucous membranes of the sinus cavities.

INTERVENTIONS

There certainly are pathogenic and hereditary factors that cause this ailment, but most headaches can be soothed, abated, and even eliminated by a long-term course of body-mind-spirit therapies. A full gamut of stress reduction therapies supplemented by a farsighted nutrition therapy program can break the headache cycle. The B-complex vitamins, especially niacin, are important in maintaining normal dilation of the cerebral blood vessels. Iron, pantothenic acid, and vitamin A have proved helpful to some people. The minerals calcium, zinc, magnesium, and potassium and the amino acid tryptophan have helped migraine sufferers.

Hemorrhoids

THE PROBLEM

These ruptured or distended veins located around the ring of the anus are unseen but felt by the sufferer. Hemorrhoids can be caused by improper lifting or by pregnancy, but more often than not, they are caused by lifestyle and nutritional factors. Diets too low in roughage and water and too high in slow-moving fats and protein foods play a major role. Poor diet, a sedentary life, and excess body weight can be common causes for hemorrhoids.

INTERVENTIONS

Hemorrhoids can be avoided and in some cases completely reversed with proper nutrition, exercise, hygiene, weight management, and improved elimination patterns. Dietary intake should include high-fiber foods, six to eight glasses of water per day, and the Reference Daily Intakes (RDIs or DRIs) of vitamins A, C, E, and B-complex.

Indigestion

THE PROBLEM

Dyspepsia is incomplete digestion that manifests in the symptoms of distension, heartburn, abdominal cramps, gas, and occasional nausea. Although it can sometimes be attributed to bacterial contamination of food, it is frequently the result of what and how we eat. Overeating, gulping air with meals, or eating during times of psychological distress can induce dyspepsia. Smoking during meals or overconsumption of gastric irritants such as coffee, tea, chocolate, or alcohol are also causative factors. Drinking copious quantities of fluids immediately before or while eating can cause indigestion. Too much fluid around mealtimes may dilute essential hydrochloric acid in the stomach and result in decreased digestive enzymes, which are necessary to digest the food.

INTERVENTIONS

How you eat is important in preventing this condition. Eat slowly, drink minimally during meals, and chew thoroughly while ingesting healing foods. Wait until you are in or induce a joyful state of mind-spirit before beginning your meal. Papaya or its commercial extract contains one of the important enzymes that aids in protein digestion in the stomach. An herbal peppermint tea can also soothe the digestive tract and stimulate digestive secretions.

Leg Cramps

THE PROBLEM

Involuntary spasms of muscles in the leg or foot most commonly occur at night and are most frequent in the young, elderly, and persons with arteriosclerosis. In the case of the elder with arteriosclerosis, it is difficult to alleviate leg cramps without surgery. In the absence of arteriosclerosis, the most common cause of leg cramps is a calcium deficiency. In some cases, a sodium loss incurred through heavy perspiration or diarrhea may be the causative factor.

INTERVENTIONS

The RDAs for vitamins B, C, and B-complex should be followed to maintain muscle strength. In addition, sufficient quantities of the minerals calcium and magnesium need to be maintained. Remember, too, that protein rebuilds damaged tissues.

Nail Problems

THE PROBLEM

Unhealthy fingernails or toenails may be the result of local injury, pathophysiology, or nutrient deficiency. Because nails are composed almost entirely of protein, suspect this area of the diet first.

INTERVENTIONS

Dietary treatment includes protein and vitamins A and B-complex. B-complex deficiencies result in fragile nails with horizontal or vertical ridges. Lack of vitamin A or calcium can cause dryness or brittleness. Frequent hangnails indicate inadequate quantities of vitamin C, folic acid, and protein. Nailbed white spots indicate zinc deficiency.

Overweight and Obesity

THE PROBLEM

Over 50 percent of American adults and 25 percent of the country's teenagers are overweight. This reversible condition contributes to all the major illnesses, including heart disease, diabetes, kidney disorders, and psychological problems. Few people, if any, are overweight on purpose. This is indeed a disorder of benign self-neglect.

INTERVENTIONS

This condition can be corrected by conscious awakening and attending to one's body-mind-spirit needs. Refer to Chapter 18 for more information on effective dieting.

Stress

THE PROBLEM

The increased production of adrenal hormones that occurs with stress increases the metabolism of protein, fats, and carbohydrates necessary to produce instant energy for the body to use to combat the perceived stressor. As a result of this increased metabolism, there is also an increased excretion of the minerals potassium, phosphorus, and calcium. Vitamin C is used by the adrenals, so if the stress is sufficiently severe or prolonged, there will be a depletion of this vitamin in the tissues. Many of the disorders related to stress are not the result of the stressor itself, but rather a result of nutritional deficiencies caused by increased metabolic rate during this period of time.

INTERVENTIONS

If you are experiencing stress, you must pay special attention to a well-balanced diet and replace the nutrients and especially B vitamins depleted during this time.

Tics, Tremors, and Twitches

THE PROBLEM

These potentially embarrassing disorders may result from ineffective coping with stress or they may be directly related to an imbalance of minerals in the body. The most common cause is a deficiency of potassium and/or magnesium. These minerals are essential for the conduction of nerve impulses that pass to a muscle and control its movement. Sometimes the B-complex vitamins, which are related to health of the nervous system, are found to be deficient. When the deficiency is corrected with supplements or B-rich foods, the symptoms may disappear. Twitches are occasionally caused by an increase of lead in the body or an allergic reaction to an allergen.

Tooth and Gum Disorders

THE PROBLEM

Dental caries can ruin an otherwise pretty smile. Most cavities are caused by persistent eating of refined sugars and starches that, when mixed with saliva, form an acid that erodes tooth enamel. Although cavities are the major dental disease, periodontitis is the ailment that causes the loss of teeth. This condition begins with gingivitis in which the gums swell, redden, and tend to bleed. Left untreated, this can lead to pyorrhea, which is characterized by further gum inflammation, recession, and loosening of teeth.

INTERVENTIONS

To prevent this condition, you must practice proper oral hygiene and eat right. All vitamins and minerals are essential, with vitamins A and C being critical. Vitamin A regulates the development and general health of the gums, while vitamin C is important for maintaining healthy gums. The minerals sodium, potassium, calcium, phosphorus, iron, and magnesium are also needed.

The preceding ailments are a sampling of what can happen when we become so busy that we forget to take care of ourselves. The good news is that most of these conditions can be reversed with conscientious nutritional self-care.

CURRENT RESEARCH STUDY

Age-Related Macular Degeneration (ARMD or AMD)

THE PROBLEM

Age-related macular degeneration (ARMD) is the leading cause of irreversible blindness in people over the age of 65, and the prevalence of ARMD is expected to increase as the population ages. The central area of the retina, primarily responsible for straight ahead and color vision, called the macula. With age, tissues break down and fluids begin to seep between the "pigment" and "transparent" layers of the retina, causing them to separate, and thus resulting in macular degeneration. The result is blurred and distorted central vision, blind spots, and loss of color vision. Although the incidence of ARMD increases sharply with age, recent studies indicate that prevention measures and dietary changes, implemented early in life, can reduce an individual's risk of ARMD. Several dietary components have been proposed and studied with regard to their ability to protect against ARMD, including antioxidant vitamins and specific carotenoids. Structural and clinical studies have shown that these carotenoids are concentrated in the retinal macular pigment and that such accumulation depends on dietary intake. Further studies have indicated that the density of the macular pigment is related to preservation of visual sensitivity and possibly protection from ARMD (Pratt, 1999). While lifestyle modifications such as smoking cessation, reduction of alcohol consumption, and wearing sunglasses may reduce the risk of ARMD, it is likely that consumption of specific dietary components can reduce the risk further.

The classic study that awakened interest in this condition evaluated the relationships between dietary intake of carotenoids and vitamins A, C, and E and the risk of ARMD. At five ophthalmology centers in the United States, 356 individuals age 55 to 80 who were diagnosed with advanced stage ARMD were studied. The 520 control subjects had other ocular diseases, and were matched to cases according to age and sex. Their relative risk for ARMD was estimated according to dietary indicators of antioxidant status, controlling for smoking and other risk factors. Analysis found that higher dietary intake of carotenoids was associated with a lower risk for ARMD. Adjusting for other risk factors, researchers found that those with the highest carotenoid intake had a 43 percent lower risk for ARMD compared to those with the lowest intake. Among the specific carotenoids, lutein and zeaxanthin, which are primarily obtained from dark green, leafy vegetables, were most strongly associated with a reduced risk for ARMD. In particular, a higher frequency of intake of spinach or collard greens was associated with a substantially lower risk for ARMD. The intake of preformed vitamin A (retinol) was not appreciably related to ARMD. Neither vitamin E nor total vitamin C consumption was associated with a statistically significant reduced risk for ARMD, although an apparently reduced risk was suggested among those with higher intake of vitamin C, particularly from foods (Seddon et al., 1994). What we do know is that increasing the consumption of foods rich in certain carotenoids, in particular dark green, leafy vegetables, may decrease the risk of developing advanced or exudative ARMD, the most visually disabling form of macular degeneration among older people.

Inverse associations have been reported between the incidence of advanced, neovascular (ARMD) and the combined lutein (L) and zeaxanthin (Z) intake in the diet and L and Z concentration in the blood serum. Research suggests that persons with high levels of L and Z in either the diet or serum would probably have, in addition, relatively high densities of these carotenoids in the macula, the so-called macular pigment. Evidence points to a potential protective effect by the macular pigment against ARMD (Bone, Landrum, Dixon, Chen, & Llerena, 2000). Epidemiological studies of diet and environmental and behavioral risk factors suggest that oxidative stress is a contributing factor to ARMD. Pathological studies indicate that damage to the retinal pigment epithelium (RPE) is an early event in ARMD. In-vitro studies show that oxidant-treated RPE cells undergo apoptosis, a possible mechanism by which RPE cells are lost during early phase of ARMD (Cai, Nelson, Wu, Sternberg, & Jones, 2000).

Evaluating 19 subjects, one study examined the relationship between dietary intake of L and Z using a food frequency questionnaire, concentration of L and Z in blood serum determined by high-performance liquid chromatography, and macular pigment optical density obtained by flicker photometry. Researchers also analyzed the serum and retinas, as autopsy samples, from 23 tissue donors in order to obtain the concentration of L and Z in these tissues. Results showed a positive, though weak, association between dietary intake of L and Z and serum concentration of L and Z, and between serum concentration of L and Z and macular pigment density. Researchers estimate that approximately half of the variability in the subjects' serum concentration of L and Z can be explained by their dietary intake of L and Z, and about one third of the variability in their macular pigment density can be attributed to their serum concentration of L and Z. These results, together with the reported associations between risk of ARMD and dietary and serum L and Z, support the hypothesis that low concentrations of macular pigment may be associated with an increased risk of ARMD (Bone et al., 2000).

Another study assessed whether dietary intake of fat or fish is associated with age-related maculopathy (ARM) prevalence. Over 3,600 people age 49 and older with ARM were identified from masked grading of retinal photographs. A 145-item, self-administered, semiquantitative food frequency questionnaire was completed adequately by 88.8 percent of participants and was used to assess intakes of dietary fat and fish. A higher frequency of fish consumption was associated with decreased odds of late ARM. Subjects with higher energy-adjusted intakes of cholesterol were significantly more likely to have late ARM, with an increased risk for late ARM for the highest compared with the lowest intake. Thus, the amount and type of dietary fat intake may be associated with ARM (Smith, Mitchell, & Leeder, 2000).

MAKING A COMMITMENT TO RESEARCH THE LINKS

Biochemical, physiological, and epidemiological research on common and uncommon applications of disease prevention takes money. Such research often requires food frequency intake evaluation and application of physiological measures to evaluate an alteration in diet and/or supplementation. There are multiple opportunities for intervention in the age-related diseases of cataract, macular degeneration, and glaucoma. These include maximizing health potential with food choice, the use of supplementation in high-risk and noncompliant patients, avoiding toxins such as cigarettes, and encouraging exercise. Economic incentives are required to explore new paradigms in nutritional preventative eye care (Richer, 2000).

ILLNESS AND DISEASE

How fortunate we are in the 21st century to understand many of the truths concerning the relationship between nutrition and disease. Today it seems hard to believe it was only a couple of generations ago that Americans suffered from debilitating diseases such as rickets, beriberi, pellagra, and scurvy. Thanks to nutritional researchers who unraveled these axioms, such gross-deficiency diseases are now understood, and because we know they can be prevented with food, these diseases are rarely found today. This is not to say, however, that nutritional diseases have been eradicated. Unfortunately, inhabitants in many Third World countries and some Americans still succumb to the ravages of these maladies.

People in developed nations may not have kwashiorkor or have their teeth fall out because of scurvy, but that does not mean that we do not suffer from other, less obvious effects of deficient diets. Actually, very few of us are as vibrantly healthy as we might be. About one-third of us will develop heart disease and one in five will die of cancer. Millions of us require medication for anxiety, depression, or pain to suppress or control the ravages of chronic diseases. Three out of 10 women will develop osteoporosis after menopause, while some 40 percent of men will develop prostate trouble. Although we may feel well enough to function and meet basic needs, we may be one of the masses who is on the borderline when it comes to living a truly healthy lifestyle.

The more we learn about the fascinating science of nutrition the more we begin to understand the incredibly important relationship between what we eat and how we feel. The following list names diseases that are still with us, some of which are on the increase. Each of the ailments may be categorized as a major disease and each of them is in some way related to nutrition. Overall well-being can be helped by an adequate diet for sufferers of these diseases. The important concept to understand is that each of these diseases can be positively affected by nutritional realignment.

Alcoholism	Diabetes
Anemia	Diverticulitis
Arteriosclerosis and atherosclerosis	Decubiti
	Gallstones
Arthritis	Gastritis
Asthma	Gout
Bronchitis	Heart disease
Bursitis	Hepatitis
Cancer	Herpes Simplex
Cataracts	Hypertension
Celiac disease	Intestinal parasites
Cirrhosis	Kidney diseases and renal stones
Colitis	Macular degeneration
Conjunctivitis	Mental illness
Cystitis	

Mononucleosis   Psoriasis

Neuritis   Pyorrhea

Osteoporosis   Rheumatic fever

Pancreatitis   Rheumatism

Parkinson's disease   Rickets

Pellagra   Sciatica

Pernicious anemia   Scurvy

Phlebitis   Shingles (herpes zoster)

Pneumonia   Sinusitis

Polio

SUMMARY

Most of the prevailing chronic diseases in the world have an important nutritional component; nutritional factors may cause a specific disease, enhance risk, exert a beneficial effect in decreasing risk, or even prevent the disease. International studies have shown that a given disease may have vastly different incidence and mortality as a function of geography. Laboratory research in animal models can reproduce fairly accurately what is learned through international research and provide the basis for examining relevant hypotheses and, more importantly, proposed actions. Research findings provide the basis for public health recommendations and health promotion activities. Through such techniques, it has been found that regular intake of foods with saturated fats such as meat and certain dairy products raise the risk of coronary heart disease. The total mixed-fat intake is associated with a higher incidence of the nutritionally linked cancers, specifically cancer of the postmenopausal breast, distal colon, prostate, pancreas, ovary, and endometrium. The associated genotoxic carcinogens for several of these cancers are heterocyclic amines, which also play a role in heart disease; they are produced during the broiling and frying of creatinine-containing foods such as meats. Monounsaturated oils such as olive or canola oil are low-risk fats as shown in animal models and through the observation that the incidence of specific diseases is lower in the Mediterranean region, where such oils are customarily used. High salt intake is associated with high blood pressure and with stomach cancer, especially with inadequate intake of potassium from fruits and vegetables and of calcium from certain vegetables and low-fat dairy products. Vegetables, fruits, and soy products are rich in antioxidants that are essential to lower disease risk stemming from reactive oxygen systems in the body. Green and black teas are excellent sources of antioxidants of a polyphenol nature, as are cocoa and some chocolates. Nutritional lifestyles that offer the possibility of a long healthy life can be adopted by most populations in the world (Weisburger, 2000). These scientific facts and figures provide us with the data we need to function as knowledgeable, professional healers.

Health care professionals have the unique opportunity to enlighten those persons with whom they come in contact in their day-to-day practices. We have the ability to empower masses of people to recognize that how, what, where, why, with whom, and when we eat makes a difference in our lives. However, we must first care for ourselves to become walking, talking, living examples of vibrant health. Only then will we be in fit condition to lead others.

REFERENCES

Bone, R. A., Landrum, J. T., Dixon, Z., Chen, Y., & Llerena, C. M. (2000). Lutein and zeaxanthin in the eyes, serum, and diet of human subjects. *Experimental Eye Research, 71*(3), 239–245.

Cai, J., Nelson, K. C., Wu, M., Sternberg, P. Jr., & Jones, D. P. (2000). Oxidative damage and protection of the RPE. *Progress in Retinal and Eye Research, 19*(2), 205–221.

Pratt, S. (1999). Dietary prevention of age-related macular degeneration. *Journal of the American Optometrists Association, 70*(1), 39–47.

Richer, S. (2000). Nutritional influences on eye health. *Optometry, 71*(10), 657–666.

Seddon, J. M., Ajani, U. A., Sperduto, R. D., Hiller, R., Blair, N., Burton, T. C., Farber, M. D., Gragoudas, E. S., Haller, J., Miller, D. T., et al. (1994). Dietary carotenoids, vitamins A, C, and E, and advanced age-related macular degeneration. Eye Disease Case-Control Study Group. *JAMA, 272*(18), 1413–1420.

Smith, W., Mitchell, P., & Leeder, S. R. (2000). Dietary fat and fish intake and age-related maculopathy. *Archives of Ophthalmology, 118*(3), 401–404.

Weisburger, J. H. (2000). Eat to live, not live to eat. *Nutrition, 16*(9), 767–773.

PART II

Understanding the Basics

CHAPTER 4

Basic Nutritional Needs

It is elevating to think of our bodies as temples for our souls. Temples, like ordinary buildings, require continual attention to ensure firm, long-standing, vital structures. In order to build and maintain strong, resilient frames in which to house our souls, we should know about our bodies' fundamental needs and how best to meet them. Human organisms are collections of bones, muscles, organs, tissues, and cells. All of these structures are composed of chemicals that come directly from the foods we eat. Human beings are remarkable creatures endowed with physical, mental, and spiritual properties that can only be actualized by an adequate intake of nourishment. The nourishment we need is multifaceted, but it includes the nutritional intake of the earth's good foods. Figure 4–1 depicts the composition of the human body in terms of chemical nutrients.

NUTRITIONAL TERMS

Some of the most common nutritional terms are defined as follows:

Nutrition—the process by which living things utilize food for energy, growth, development, and maintenance. We eat foods to provide nutrients for necessary body functions and to make essential compounds. Many of these nutrients cannot be synthesized, so we must obtain them in our daily food. Nutrition involves digesting foods and absorbing and delivering nutrients to the cells where they are utilized. It also includes picking up and carrying the waste products to the bloodstream.

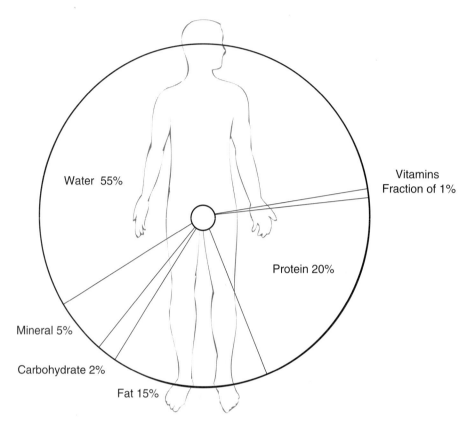

Figure 4–1 Approximate nutrient composition of the human body.

Food—any substance ingested into the body to provide nutrients.

Gram—a unit of weight. Most food labels list contents in terms of grams. For many foods, 30 grams equals 1 ounce.

Health—the state of optimal physical, mental, spiritual, and social well-being.

Nutrients—biochemical substances used by the body. The six major classes of nutrients obtained from foods are water, protein, carbohydrates, fats, minerals, and vitamins.

Malnutrition—a condition that arises from a prolonged lack of or excessive intake of nutrients or an impaired utilization of food.

Megadose—a quantity of a vitamin or mineral that exceeds by 10 times or more the daily recommended intake of that substance.

Recommended Dietary Allowances (RDAs)—a measure of nutritional needs in terms of specific amounts of nutrients that a healthy individual should receive every day. These nutrients help us achieve full growth and development potential. RDAs were intended to be desirable daily amounts of nutrients to be consumed by healthy people. This term was introduced in 1973 as a reference value for vitamins, minerals, and protein in voluntary nutritional labeling. In 1992, the term was renamed *Reference Daily Intakes* (RDIs; also sometimes referred to as DRIs). Despite the name change, the actual values (except for the value of protein) remain the same.

Daily Reference Values (DRVs)—figures for nutrients such as fat and cholesterol for which no standards previously existed. The figures are based on the number of calories consumed per day. For labeling purposes, 2,000 calories has been established as the reference for calculating percent daily values. Whatever the caloric level, DRVs for the energy-producing nutrients are always calculated as follows:

- fat based on 30 percent of calories
- saturated fat based on 10 percent of calories
- carbohydrates based on 60 percent of calories
- protein based on 10 percent of calories
- fiber based on 11.5 grams of fiber per 1,000 calories

The DRVs for cholesterol, sodium, and potassium, which do not contribute calories, remain the same regardless of the calorie level. Table 4–1 shows DRVs of the major food components.

TABLE 4–1 Daily Reference Values (DRVs)*, Reference Daily Intakes (RDIs or DRIs)

FOOD COMPONENT	DRV
Fat	65 grams
Saturated fatty acids	20 grams
Cholesterol	300 milligrams
Total carbohydrate	300 grams
Fiber	25 grams
Sodium	2,400 milligrams
Potassium	2,400 milligrams
Protein**	50 grams

*Based on 2,000 calories a day for adults and children over 4 years old
**DRV for protein does not apply to certain populations; DRI for protein has been established for these groups: children 1 to 4 years: 16 grams; infants under a year: 14 grams; pregnant women: 60 grams; and nursing women: 65 grams.

Source: *FDA Consumer,* May 1993.

WATER AND CHEMICALS

Water

Cosmic dust swirled from the universe and settled in the Milky Way galaxy billions of years ago to form planet Earth. Water, the liquid from which life arose, was probably locked into rock-forming compounds. These compounds slowly released the trapped water during the first billion years or so of Earth's history and formed the primordial oceans. Water became the most common substance on Earth and now covers more than 70 percent of the planet's surface. From the primordial saline oceans, living, breathing organisms arose, and from those organisms came human life. All living things consist mostly of water; our bodies are about two-thirds water. Because so much of our physical being is fluid, we need to keep recycling our systems with clean, fresh water. We are advised to drink six to eight glasses of pure water each day because we need to continually renew our body fluids.

Just as the ocean provides tremendous means of transportation for the cargo of goods distributed worldwide, the fluid in our arteries and veins serves as the transportation system for the whole of our bodies. Oceans clearly play an essential role in life on Earth, yet because of their vastness, humans have used their waters as dumping grounds for many waste materials. Just as we must not allow our oceans to become polluted, so too we must keep our bodies clean by replenishing them with clean, pure water. Waste materials and toxins need daily flushings to maintain homeostasis. Homeostasis, which is standard for any healthy organism, involves the maintenance of a steady state within a biological system by means of self-regulating mechanisms.

Chemical Composition

The human body is made up of numerous chemical elements, but the main components are oxygen, hydrogen, carbon, and nitrogen. These elements, which are derived directly or indirectly from the atmosphere or from water, account for nearly 95 percent of total body weight. The remaining elements include:

1. the minerals calcium and phosphorus, which, as constituents of bone, account for about another 3 percent of body weight.
2. in order of decreasing amounts: potassium, sodium, magnesium, iron, zinc, and copper.
3. several trace elements such as vanadium, chromium, silicon, and selenium.

On the molecular level, the body's chemicals are organized into two major categories: inorganic and organic compounds. Organic compounds are the carbon-containing compounds, the main types of which include proteins, lipids (fats), and carbohydrates. Each of these compounds is discussed in detail in other chapters. Water constitutes roughly 60 percent of total body weight and is essential for almost all chemical reactions within the body.

The molecular constituents of the body are combined to form cells and extracellular materials. The adult human body contains approximately 100 trillion cells, which are organized and differentiated to form a number of different kinds of tissues with specific functions. We can affect these trillions of cells with healing nutrition. Because we are constantly shedding old cells and developing new ones, we have the opportunity to build new cells with the best nutritional elements and compounds available.

It is from our cells that we build the four main types of tissue: epithelial, muscle, nerve, and connective. Epithelial tissue, which covers the body's surface and lines its tubes, protects these surfaces. Epithelial tissue is the site of various absorption and excretion processes. Also included in epithelial tissue are the outgrowths and ingrowths that form the surfaces of sensory organs, glands, hair, nails, and other structures. Muscle tissue enables the body to move through its ability to contract and relax. Nerve tissue, made up of neurons, conducts information signals and processes data. Connective tissue, which contains large amounts of extracellular matter, provides support for the body in the form of tendons, ligaments, cartilage, bone, and fat deposits. Lastly, blood and lymph are fluids that are sometimes also considered as tissues. Together they convey nutrients, waste products, and the specialized defensive cells of the immune system through the different parts of the body.

CALORIC REQUIREMENTS

For the most part, Americans consume more calories than we need. Caloric requirements depend on your size, age, and level of activity. Table 4–2 (on page 48) shows some approximate daily caloric needs.

Foods vary markedly in their caloric values. When attempting to stay within a range of caloric consumption, it is important to know which foods will add substantial calories to our intake. Table 4–3 (on page 48) lists common foods and the calories they provide.

DIETARY FIBER

Dietary fiber includes all food substances that our digestive enzymes cannot break down. Since we cannot digest fiber, it is not used by the body as an energy source. There are six major types of dietary fiber:

1. *Cellulose* is the major constituent of plant fiber, found in the plant cell walls.
2. *Hemicellulose* is closely associated with the cell walls of plants.

TABLE 4–2 — Basic Caloric Requirements

NUMBER OF CALORIES	BODY TYPE, AGE, AND LEVEL OF ACTIVITY
1,600	Sedentary women
	Some older adults
2,200	Most children
	Teenage girls
	Active women (pregnant or lactating women may need more)
	Sedentary men
2,800	Teenage boys
	Most active men
	Very active women
3,000 and up	Athletes in training

TABLE 4–3 — Caloric Content of Common Foods

ITEM	AMOUNT	CALORIES
Cottage cheese	1 cup	225
Mozzarella	1 ounce	90
American cheese	1 ounce	105
Sour cream	1 cup	230
Yogurt (flavored, whole milk)	1 cup	260
Yogurt (skim milk)	1 cup	127
Boiled egg	1	80
Fried egg	1	85
Butter	1 stick	865
Fish (baked)	3 ounces	135
Crab meat	1 cup	135
Tuna meat (oil packed)	1 cup	295
Tuna meat (water packed)	1 cup	160
Bacon	2 slices	85
Beef (very lean)	3 ounces	245
Ham (lean)	3 ounces	245
Chicken breast	2.8 ounces	160
Apple	1	80
Avocado	1	370
Banana	1	100
Bread	1 loaf	1,195
Bread	1 slice	65
Chocolate chip cookies	4	200
Macaroni and cheese	1 cup	430
Walnuts	1 cup	785
Green beans (frozen)	1 cup	35
Corn (frozen)	1 cup	134

3. *Lignin* is a woody compound found not only in wood but also in plant fibers.
4. *Pectin* is found in roots, stems, and fruits of plants, especially in apples and citrus rinds, and is famous for its jelling properties.
5. *Gums* and *mucilage* occur naturally in foods such as guar and legumes, and are used in many prepared food products.
6. *Algal polysaccharides* are gel-forming fibers found in sea vegetables, including kelp, kombu, carrageenan, and agar.

Each of the six types of fibers fit into one of two basic categories: water insoluble (which do not dissolve in water) and water soluble (which mix with water). Insoluble fibers such as those found in cellulose, hemicellulose, and lignin stimulate the intestines, decrease food transit time, and increase the weight and softness of the stool. Insoluble fiber is found in wheat bran, whole grains, fruits, vegetables, and nuts.

The soluble fibers of pectin, gums, mucilages, algal polysaccharides, and certain hemicelluloses are found in fruits, oats, barley, legumes, psyllium, seeds, flax seeds, and sea vegetables. Responsible for most beneficial effects of fiber, these soluble fibers lower the absorption of cholesterol, regulate the blood sugar by slowing the absorption of sugar into the bloodstream, and absorb and remove toxic materials and carcinogens from the body. Although they are important to all of us, soluble fibers are of special interest to individuals with diabetes because these fibers keep the blood sugar at a more constant level. Hypoglycemia may be treated by using the slow sugar absorption properties of soluble fibers. Insoluble fibers, however, do not stabilize the blood sugar in the same way.

Wheat bran is one of the least expensive ways to obtain insoluble fiber. Wheat bran is easily added to breads, casseroles, soups, and cereals. Because it is extremely high in insoluble fibers, wheat bran accelerates transit time more than most foods by acting as an irritant to the intestines. Wheat bran must be used with large amounts of water to prevent cramping, flatulence, or constipation. Unlike soluble fibers, wheat bran increases the absorption rate of sugars into the bloodstream which may cause adverse blood sugar fluctuations in hypoglycemic and diabetic conditions. Since it is high in mineral-binding phytic acid, which binds minerals and makes them unavailable for the body to absorb, wheat bran should be used in moderation.

Oat bran, an excellent soluble fiber noted for its use in lowering cholesterol, is as effective as other soluble fibers. Like wheat bran, oat bran can be added to breads, casseroles, soups, and cereals, or it can be made into a cooked cereal. Its lighter color, texture, and flavor make it even more appealing than wheat bran. Since it contains some natural oils, it should be refrigerated or stored in the freezer for no more than two months.

Flax seeds are most commonly used as a healthy addition to breads and baked goods. The outer walls of the seeds swell and absorb water to form a mucilage coating that provides bulk and lubrication.

Guar gum, which is often found listed on the labels of commercially prepared whipped cream products, is a mucilaginous substance derived from legumes. Guar gum acts in a similar fashion to pectin.

Pectin, which is found in apples, is purified and used in antidiarrhea preparations. It is also used when making jams and jellies. It forms a jellylike substance and has all the beneficial effects of other soluble fibers.

Psyllium seeds are similar to flax seeds and are derived from the plantago plant. Most are used for their fiber-rich husks. The outer walls of the seeds swell and absorb water to form a mucilage coating that provides bulk and lubrication. Because psyllium seeds swell so rapidly, preparations made with them should be used immediately. Psyllium seeds have been used in many commercial laxatives for years.

How Much Fiber Do We Need?

The average low-fiber, refined diet provides about 10 to 20 grams of fiber per day. The conservative RDI quantity is 25 to 35 grams per day, but suggested optimal amounts range from 30 to 50 grams per day. Any increase should be gradual in order to give the digestive system time to adjust. The amount of water taken in needs to be increased as well.

To increase fiber intake, start by eating a bran muffin instead of a croissant and brown rice instead of white rice. Do not peel vegetables unless they are waxed or have suffered surface damage, but be sure to wash them thoroughly. Eat whole fruit instead of drinking the juice. Generally, counting grams of fiber is not necessary if high-fiber substitutions are made. When reading food tables and labels, look for the words *dietary fiber* instead of *crude fiber*. Dietary fiber includes all the different fibers present in a food.

ADJUSTING TO INCREASED FIBER

Increasing fiber intake may cause:

- *Digestive discomforts.* Common reactions to increased fiber in the diet are flatulence and bloating. However, both can be minimized if proper precautions are taken. Gradually increasing fiber intake will decrease these symptoms. This means adding just one serving of a high-fiber food daily for a week. The next week, add another serving per day. Make ongoing diet changes that include high-fiber foods rather than processed, low-fiber foods. The second important step is to increase liquid intake to about 8 to 10 glasses of water per day to account for the extra liquid that will be absorbed by the fiber. This is the real key for the effectiveness of fiber. Too little liquid combined with more fiber intake can cause constipation, and possibly an intestinal blockage.

- *Mineral deficiencies.* Too much fiber may lead to mineral deficiencies because fiber compounds, especially phytic acid and oxalic acid, bind with minerals to block absorption. However, mineral-binding phytic acid can be destroyed if high-fiber grains, nuts, and legumes are cooked, fermented, sprouted, or made into a yeast-risen bread.
- *Changes in the body's use of medications in certain illnesses.* Individuals with specific medical conditions, especially diabetes, hypoglycemia, and elevated cholesterol, should discuss an increase in fiber with their doctor, dietitian, or qualified health professional. Increased fiber may reduce the need for insulin and other medications.

High-Fiber Foods

Because all fiber sources except lignin are complex carbohydrates, the best way to increase fiber in the diet is to eat whole foods that are high in complex carbohydrates. Overprocessed foods like white flour, white sugar, and white rice are low in fiber and in other nutrients. Canned fruits and vegetables are much lower in fiber than their fresh whole or frozen counterparts. Overcooking also reduces the amount of available fiber. Try to include both insoluble and soluble fibers in your diet. Table 4–4 details the fiber content of some foods.

HEALTH CARE PROVIDER ROLES REGARDING NUTRITION

To be effective practitioners, we need to know facts and figures to support our scientific knowledge base. Despite the power of data and numbers, we need more. As human beings striving to actualize our human potentials and helping others reach theirs, we need information that motivates us, stirs our psyche, and awakens our dreams. For many, it is the hope or dream of a better life or release from the clutches of illness or disease that motivates change. Health care providers encounter clients in every conceivable life circumstance. Armed with nutrition information and knowledge of how to stimulate motivation for lifestyle change, we can help clients realize the power of healthy nutrition. Specific clinical roles include counseling or guidance in the following areas:

- lifestyle behavioral changes
- general nutrition
- eating disorders
- special clinical diets: diabetes, cancer, and heart disease
- maternal, child, and elder nutrition
- weight reduction and weight management programs

TABLE 4-4	**Fiber Content in Selected Foods**	

FOOD	SERVING	GRAMS OF DIETARY FIBER
Whole wheat bread	1 slice	2.6
White bread	1 slice	0.63
Granola	½ cup	6.4
Oatmeal	½ cup, cooked	2.1
Popcorn	1 cup	1.3
Brown rice	½ cup, cooked	3.7
White rice	½ cup, cooked	1.5
Black beans	½ cup, cooked	7.7
Almonds	¼ cup, whole	4.4
Broccoli	½ cup, cooked	5.5
Carrot	1 medium, raw	2.3
Kale (without stems)	1 cup, cooked	3.5
Lettuce (loose leaf)	1 cup, chopped	0.8
Peas, frozen	½ cup, cooked	3.6
Potato (med.)	1 baked in peel	4.7
Winter squash	1 cup, baked	6.9
Apple	1 medium	3.5
Banana	1 fresh	2.3
Figs	2 medium, dried	4.0
Orange	1 medium	3.1
Orange juice	1 cup, fresh	1.0
Peach	1 medium	1.5

Teamwork is effective in many areas of healing; nutrition is no exception. When providing guidance to clients, rely on the help and support of dietitians, nutritionists, and other healing professionals.

FOOD MISINFORMATION

It is important to note that although traditional nutrition, like everything else "traditional," is undergoing a revolution, there is still much valuable information in our basic textbooks. Although this book includes some often neglected information such as living foods and vegetarianism, it does not negate the adequacy of numerous basic nutrition guides. When studying nutrition, it is important not to fall prey to food faddist claims of panaceas. Often food faddists include one or more of the following claims in their conversations:

1. Only certain foods will cure your condition.
2. Certain foods are harmful and should be eliminated from your diet.

3. Particular food combinations have special therapeutic effects.

4. You may be vitamin or mineral deficient if you do not measure up to their muscle-testing method.

5. Only natural foods or vitamins can meet nutritional needs and prevent disease.

All or any one of these claims should make you suspicious. Healthy nutrition is not about eliminating or adding any one product to your diet. It is about discovering and maintaining balance with all food groups as you simultaneously balance your mind and spirit.

Unscientific information about food can mislead you and your clients and contribute to poor food habits and a rapidly dwindling bank account. False information may be based on subtle half-truths, innuendos, or outright deception. Food faddists appeal to vulnerable groups such as the elderly and overweight people. Figure-conscious people or those with an exaggerated idea of glamour can fall prey to flashy advertisements that offer crash programs to achieve the ideal weight, muscle strength, beauty, or vitality. The best protection against food charlatans is to augment your knowledge of healing nutrition. Practice it and teach it to your clients. Remember, as much as we have come to respect our intuitive abilities, professional practice is based in science. When clients ask us to evaluate a nutritional program, we need to teach them the value of asking significant questions. They, in turn, should ask these questions of diet or food promoters.

1. What is the program about?
2. What is the rationale for the program?
3. What is your evidence?
4. How does the program work?

CASE STUDY: Elizabeth

Elizabeth was a 17-year-old high school junior. She struggled to be a high achiever and studied conscientiously for her finals and for the Scholastic Aptitude Test (SAT). She knew that if she could maintain her 3.6 grade point average (GPA), and score over 1,200 on the SAT, she would be eligible for a college scholarship that could make all the difference in her life.

Elizabeth was first seen at the end of June by a health professional at one of the city emergency rooms. Her primary complaint was that her mouth was sore and her gums were bleeding. She had a temperature of 101°F and felt tired and listless. The young doctor in the emergency room

(Continued on next page)

told her she probably had some sort of virus but prescribed antibiotics just in case it was a bacterial infection. Three days later, when she felt no better and her teeth began to feel loose, her mother took her to a health practitioner who had special evening clinic sessions at the high school.

When the practitioner questioned Elizabeth about dietary intake, she learned that in addition to being under tremendous stress regarding her academic achievement, Elizabeth was dieting. Elizabeth had lost 20 pounds during the past 6 weeks and intended to shed 10 more. She thought she had gained entirely too much weight during the academic year. Now that the school year was over, she was concentrating on weight loss, and was helping her mother move out of their home into an apartment. When the practitioner asked Elizabeth, "Do you think you may be under some stress?" the reply was immediate: "Of course I am! I never have a free minute and I worry about our new living arrangements all the time. Wouldn't you be under stress too?" In response to questions about her diet, Elizabeth said she primarily ate chicken noodle soup with occasional dill pickles for snacks. That diet had worked for some of her friends and she suspected that it would work for her too. Besides, she had heard that chicken soup was supposed to be healing.

The practitioner thought Elizabeth was probably severely nutritionally malnourished and counseled her and her mother about dietary recommendations. She also gave Elizabeth a pamphlet on stress management and referred her to a local dentist.

The dentist made the final diagnosis of scurvy. He debrided Elizabeth's mouth with pressure sprays of grapefruit juice and gave her prescriptions for lysine, vitamin C, and acidophilis. He reinforced the practitioner's instructions for long periods of rest and relaxation as he told Elizabeth that she had a disease of stress. The emotional pressure she had been under for months had undermined her vitamin C stores. Because she was dieting and not eating fruits and vegetables or taking vitamin supplements, she had no vitamin C intake. She also did not have sufficient intake of the essential amino acids to rebuild new tissues and hence developed one of humankind's oldest ailments.

Elizabeth and her mother were amazed that she had come so close to actually losing her teeth because of misguided and insufficient nutritional information. After that experience, both mother and daughter became converts to balanced nutritional eating patterns.

Observations

Elizabeth was misdiagnosed and undertreated in the hospital emergency room because the physician did not consider nutrition as a pos-

(Continued on next page)

sible cause of disease. People in good nutritional health are usually robust with bright eyes and shiny hair. Fatness or thinness is not an indication of nutritional health. Elizabeth deviated radically from healthy nutritional guidelines. When doing physical examinations and taking histories, we must remember that nutrition continues to be an important part of the overall health assessment.

SUMMARY

Good nutrition is an essential part of life, and having some knowledge about our basic needs helps us achieve good nutrition. Our bodies are composed of water and biochemicals. To feel and function at an optimal level we need the right amount of the basic calories and dietary fiber. As the field of nutrition grows so too does propaganda and misinformation about food. Sometimes in an effort to be on the leading edge of new information, data is released and/or misconstrued before scientific research validates the effectiveness of the new food or food combination. Health care providers will want to critically analyze whether new food information meets certain criteria. Getting the right assortment of biochemicals is addressed in the next few chapters.

CHAPTER 5

Proteins

COMPOSITION

Proteins, the main building blocks of cells, are large, complex molecules (macromolecules) made up of polypeptides, which in turn are made up of the nitrogen-containing amino acids. Proteins constitute about 15 percent of the body by weight, form much of the body's structure, and serve important chemical functions, particularly in the form of enzymes. Proteins are essential molecules that people must have to maintain the structure and function of a healthy body. They have many different properties and function in a variety of ways. The term *protein* is derived from the Greek word *proteios,* meaning "primary." Enzymes, hemoglobin, certain hormones, and the collagen in bones, tendons, and skin are all proteins.

Proteins exist in diverse, complex structures that specify their particular function. The group is comprised of about 20 amino acids. Each amino acid is composed of an amino group, a carboxyl group, and a carbon side chain that specifies the characteristics of the particular amino acid. A primary protein is simply a long chain of amino acids linked together with a peptide bond between the amino group of one and the carboxyl group of another. The sequence of the amino acids in the chain varies with each type of protein. The amino acids constituting a protein are arranged in such a way as to give rise to periodic, secondary structures. The way in which a protein folds into its final conformation, or shape, is vital to its function.

CASE STUDY: Cynthia

Cynthia was a 19-year-old student who was determined to look good and feel fit as she studied to become a nurse. When she entered the program a year ago, she saw that many of her student peers and faculty were overweight and she resolved not to allow this to happen to her. She began an unmonitored, self-imposed, protein-restricted diet and remained on it for a year. She did stay slim, but as she entered her sophomore year, she began to notice some physical changes. Her hair lost its luster, her fingernails broke, and she felt tired all the time.

In her sophomore year, Cynthia took a required nutrition course. While taking this course, she learned the important role of food in health and realized that she had the symptoms of protein deficiency. She quickly modified her food intake to include adequate proteins. Within three months, her symptoms reversed and her energy returned. Cynthia was lucky. Others who are unaware of or do not realize the significance of healing nutrition can succumb to multiple diseases of omission or even premature death.

Observations

Unfortunately, Cynthia is typical of many young girls. In an effort to look svelte and be popular, many teenagers and young women sacrifice good nutrition for poor health. Lack of protein can cause patchy brown spots to appear on the skin and loss of hair. It can instigate diarrhea, anemia, vitamin deficiencies, fluid retention, and high blood pressure. Mental problems can also result from the lack of protein. Clients may experience maladies such as apathy, irritability, poor concentration, memory loss, and general fatigue. As health care providers, we need to be alert to problems of faulty nutrition in people.

PROTEIN AND DIET

Protein is a critically important part of the diet. While plants synthesize all the amino acids required for building the necessary proteins, animals do not. Humans need dietary intake to synthesize 10 essential amino acids, and therefore, are dependent on food to maintain health. Proteins help replace and form new tissue and transport nutrients in and out of cells. They regulate the balance of water, acids, and bases, and are essential in making antibodies. Proteins play a role in virtually every cellular function. For instance, proteins regulate muscle contraction and expansion and contraction of the blood vessels to maintain normal blood pressure.

The protein we eat is broken down into amino acids during digestion. These amino acids are absorbed into the bloodstream, where they travel to tissues throughout the body. Cells build up new proteins from these amino acids to serve specific functions. Generally, a lack of protein in the diet retards growth in children and causes a decrease in energy. A failure to consume adequate quantities of food energy may lead to weight loss or growth failure in children, wasting of tissues, and eventually starvation. The production of enzymes and hormones is impaired in severe protein deficiency. Young children living in poorer communities throughout the world commonly have protein-energy malnutrition (PEM). The two clinical forms of PEM are nutritional marasmus and kwashiorkor. Marasmus is due primarily to a calorie deficiency, while kwashiorkor results from a protein deficiency. Mild or moderate PEM is much more common than these two severe forms and contributes to a slow rate of growth, poor development, increased susceptibility to infections, and eventually to the potential for permanent physical stunting.

Proteins are essential as the building blocks of our cells. It is imperative that all of us know something about them. Protein, like other nutrients, can be detrimental if it is either overconsumed or underconsumed. This nutrient, like almost everything else in our lives, must be understood and used in moderation.

How Much Protein Do We Need?

This answer is much less than you may think. Most Americans eat twice as much protein as RDAs suggest, but then again, many Americans are overweight. There are times when we may need additional amounts of protein. If we are undergoing extra physical or psychological stress or recovering from infections, we may need a protein boost. Infants, growing children, and pregnant and lactating women require the most protein per pound of ideal body weight.

The National Research Council of the National Academy of Sciences considers the average adult's daily requirement to be 0.8 percent of protein for each kilogram of body weight. To determine the daily protein needs for a healthy adult, use the following formula:

Determine the weight in pounds.

Convert weight to kilograms by dividing the pounds by 2.2.

Multiply weight in kilograms by 0.8, which yields grams of protein needed by the individual.

Example: A woman who weighs 140 pounds.

$140 \div 2.2 = 63.6$ kilograms

$63.6 \times 0.8 = 50.88$ grams of protein

Calculate your daily protein needs then begin reading food labels and nutrition charts to see if you are on track. If you are overweight, calculate your protein needs based on your ideal body weight.

Can Too Much Protein Be Harmful?

Over time, too much protein can contribute to the development of heart disease, osteoporosis, obesity, kidney disease, gout, and certain forms of cancer such as breast, prostate, and colon cancer. Some of these diseases are also caused by the fact that a high protein intake is often accompanied by a high fat intake, especially in people who eat an excess of meat and milk products. In general, the average daily protein intake by adults in the United States exceeds the 0.8 to 1.6 gram per kilogram of body weight, equal to 0.36 to 0.73 grams per pound of body weight, recommended by the National Academy of Sciences. The results of one 6-year study showed that women who ate beef, pork, or lamb as a main dish every day had 2.5 times the risk of developing colon cancer as women who consumed these red meats less than once a month.

Since protein is not stored in the body, stress is put on the kidneys as they try to eliminate surplus amounts. Excess protein has long been associated with the buildup of uric acid that can result in gout. If you have ever known a heavy meat eater who suffered from a throbbing big toe, you know about gout. At the same time, excess protein increases the amount of calcium excreted, creating a potential risk for osteoporosis and kidney stones. But to top it off, excess protein may make you fat. Due to the high levels of fat and cholesterol found in many animal protein-containing foods, the National Research Council, the American Heart Association, and many health care practitioners are recommending that smaller and fewer portions of meat and high-fat cheese be eaten.

Epidemiological evidence suggests a link between meat consumption and prostate cancer. In one study, benign prostatic hyperplasia tissues were examined for CYP1 expression and for their ability to metabolically activate carcinogens found in cooked meat. Results showed that human prostate tissue can metabolically activate "cooked meat" carcinogens, a process that may contribute to prostate cancer development (Williams et al., 2000).

In heart disease, the protein cholesteryl ester transfer protein (CETP) is a plasma glycoprotein that mediates the transfer of cholesteryl ester from high-density lipoproteins (HDL) to triglyceride-rich lipoproteins in exchange for triglycerides (Ordovas, 2000). In excess, Lp(a), a lipoprotein, is an independent risk factor for recurrent atherosclerotic heart disease in men and in women after menopause. Research is being conducted on drugs to lower Lp(a); however, a low cholesterol–forming diet and other lifestyle modifications currently are the best treatments (Futterman & Lemberg, 2001).

How to Reduce Protein Intake

If you are a heavy meat eater, you may want to make a conscious effort to reduce protein intake. Begin by eliminating meat from one meal a day and using meat and poultry as a condiment rather than the entree for the second meal of the day. After a period of time, you may want to try eating meat at only one meal a day. You may want to substitute beans, lentils, tofu, and other vegetable protein sources in place of the meat and poultry. With quality meat at only one meal, you should still have sufficient intake quantities. A good rule of thumb is to limit each protein serving to 3 ounces (the size of a deck of cards) of cooked, trimmed beef, pork, lamb, poultry, or fish per meal, with a maximum of 6 ounces per day. If you want to try a meatless regime, see Chapter 14 on vegetarianism.

MEAT

Meat products include beef, veal (calves), pork, lamb, and venison (deer). Meat is both caloric and fatty. Some people select marbled beef believing it to be the tastiest. The marbling, however, connotes fat, and fat is what makes meat consumption questionable as a healthy behavior.

Buying Meat

Purchase lean meats closely trimmed of fat, or trim them yourself at home. Prime, the most heavily marbled grade of meat, has the highest fat content, followed by Choice and Select. If buying veal, ask for naturally raised veal. These calves are allowed to walk and mingle in small herds. Although it remains slightly pink after cooking, naturally raised veal has the added benefit of being more flavorful and juicy than the pale white meat from calves that are formula-fed and tethered in small, cramped quarters.

Table 5–1 depicts the various nutrients in the most popular cuts of meat.

Lean Meat Cooking Tips

Keep lean meat lean. Avoid frying; instead, bake, broil, grill, or roast on a rack. Lightly sauté or stir-fry with minimal oil. Marinate with spices, wine, or lemon instead of oil. For maximum tenderness, cook lean meats slowly with low or moderate moist heat. High heat toughens and dries meat. In particular, avoid overcooking lean cuts, which can become dry, tough, and tasteless if cooked too long.

TABLE 5–1	**Meat Nutrition Information**

BEEF, PORK, LAMB, & VEAL	Total Calories	Protein	Carbohydrates	Total Fat	Saturated Fatty Acids	Cholesterol	Sodium	Vitamin A	Vitamin C	Calcium	Iron
	KCAL	G	G	G	G	MG	MG	% U.S. RDA			
Beef											
Top round steak	216	30	0	10	4	85	60	0	0	7	3
Sirloin steak	215	29	0	10	4	89	65	0	0	11	3
Tenderloin steak	235	27	0	13	5	85	62	0	0	7	3
Top loin steak	98	29	10	8	3	76	68	0	0	8	8
Eye of round	171	29	0	5	2	69	62	0	0	5	2
Tip round	191	28	0	8	3	81	64	0	0	5	3
Bottom round	188	29	0	7	3	78	66	0	0	5	3
Chuck arm roast	280	30	0	17	7	100	62	0	0	10	3
Ground beef, extra lean	265	28	0	16	6	99	82	0	0	9	3
Ground round	292	27	0	20	8	101	93	0	0	12	3
Pork											
Center loin chop	229	30	0	11	4	81	63	6	0	29	1
Fresh whole ham	278	27	0	18	7	94	60	10	0	7	1
Shoulder picnic cut	317	23	0	24	9	94	70	8	0	19	1
Tenderloin	201	30	0	8	3	94	64	7	1	5	1
Lamb											
Leg of lamb	258	25	0	17	7	93	66	*	*	11	2
Loin chop	316	25	0	23	10	100	77	*	*	20	2
Shoulder arm chop	278	24	0	19	8	97	78	*	*	21	2
Rib roast	359	21	0	30	13	97	73	*	*	22	2
Arm chop	281	24	0	20	8	96	77	*	*	18	2
Veal											
Cutlet (top round)	211	36	0	6	3	134	67	*	*	8	1
Sirloin	252	31	0	13	5	108	79	*	*	17	1
Ground	172	24	0	8	3	103	83	*	*	17	1

Serving Size: 3.5 oz. (trimmed to 0 fat) cooked portion broiled, braised, or roasted without additional fat, sodium, or sauces.

*Indicates no available data.

Source: *USDA Agricultural Handbook.*

Storing Meat

Properly wrapped and stored, fresh steaks, chops, and roasts can be safely kept for 3 to 5 days in the refrigerator or 6 to 9 months in the freezer. Ground or stew meats and organ meats, such as heart and liver, should be used within 1 to 2 days. They may also be frozen for 3 to 4 months. Cooked meat and meat dishes can be used for leftovers for 3 to 4 days when stored in the refrigerator or 2 to 3 months in the freezer.

Keeping Meat Safe

The recent deaths and serious illnesses from tainted hamburgers underscore the importance of food safety. Most meat and poultry contain millions of bacteria, some of them quite dangerous. But through proper food handling, the bacteria can be prevented from multiplying to numbers large enough to cause illness. The following precautions should ensure safety.

1. *Cook hamburger meat thoroughly, until no pink color shows at the center of the patty.* Hamburger meat is riskier than steaks and other cuts because it is ground and mixed, giving it a much larger surface area for bacterial growth.

2. *Use a meat thermometer.* Cook all meats to an internal temperature of at least 160 degrees. Red meat is done when it is brown or gray inside. Poultry is done when its juices run clear and no pink color shows at the center or next to the bone. Rare beef does carry some bacterial risk.

3. *Wash your hands.* Wash your hands in hot, soapy water before and after handling raw meat or poultry. Wash them again during food preparation if you sneeze, cough, or blow your nose.

4. *Use separate cutting boards for preparing raw meats.* Wash cutting boards with hot, soapy water after use. Occasionally give them a second wash with a mild bleach solution and rinse with clean water.

5. *Use clean utensils.* Never use utensils that have touched raw meat and poultry without thoroughly washing them first.

6. *Use clean sponges and towels.* Clean up drippings from raw meat with a paper towel to avoid contaminating a sponge or dishcloth.

7. *Observe the "sell by" and "use by" dates.*

8. *Do not trust your nose.* Although you should not prepare meats that smell bad, do not trust your nose. You cannot smell bacteria.

9. *Never thaw meat or poultry at room temperature.* Thaw in the refrigerator or microwave oven.

10. *Do not let meat stand at room temperature for more than two hours.* Food that sits on a warming tray for a long time is especially vulnerable to bacterial growth.

11. *Store meats properly in the refrigerator.* Store raw roasts and steaks in the refrigerator no longer than 3 to 5 days, raw hamburger and stew meat no longer than 2 days, raw chicken or turkey no longer than 1 to 2 days, and leftover cooked meats no longer than 3 to 4 days.

FISH

Seafood is generally lower in calories than meat. Table 5–2 depicts the nutritional values for the 20 most commonly consumed types of seafood. Values are given for a single serving—a 3-ounce, cooked, skinless portion. Use this information to choose a healthy diet that includes a variety of seafood.

Selecting Fresh Fish

Whatever the variety, whole fish have certain characteristics that indicate freshness. Look for

- bright, clear, full eyes that are often protruding. As a fish loses freshness, the eyes become cloudy, pink, and sunken.
- firm and elastic flesh that springs back when pressed gently with the finger. With time, the flesh becomes soft and slips from the bone.
- shiny skin with scales that adhere tightly. Characteristic colors and markings start to fade as soon as the fish leaves the water.
- a clean, pink intestinal cavity.
- a fresh, mild odor.

Fillets and fish steaks should have a firm and elastic flesh and a fresh-cut appearance with no browning or drying around the edges.

Storing Fresh Fish

Fresh fish should be kept in the coldest part of the refrigerator and cooked within 1 or 2 days.

Buying Frozen Fish

The technology of handling seafood has improved tremendously in recent years. Commercially frozen fish has been quickly frozen at its peak while still on board the fishing vessel. When properly thawed, it is comparable to fish that was never frozen and exhibits the same qualities of freshness. When buying frozen fish, look for packages that still have their original shape with the wrappings intact and no visible ice or blood.

TABLE 5–2 Seafood Nutrition Information

SEAFOOD	Total Calories KCAL	Protein G	Carbohydrates G	Total Fat G	Saturated Fatty Acids G	Cholesterol MG	Sodium MG	Vitamin A % U.S. RDA	Vitamin C % U.S. RDA	Calcium % U.S. RDA	Iron % U.S. RDA
Blue Crab, steamed	90	19	0	1	0	80	310	*	*	9	4
Catfish, baked	120	19	0	5	1	60	65	*	*	3	5
Clam, steamed, 12 small	130	22	4	2	0	60	95	10	*	8	130
Cod, broiled	90	19	0	1	0	50	60	*	2	*	2
Flounder, baked	100	20	0	1	0	50	85	*	*	2	2
Haddock, baked	90	20	0	1	0	60	70	*	*	4	6
Halibut, broiled	120	22	0	2	0	30	60	3	*	5	5
Lobster, broiled	100	20	1	1	0	100	320	*	*	5	2
Mackerel, Atlantic, Pacific, & Jack, broiled	190	21	0	12	3	60	95	7	*	*	9
Mahi Mahi, broiled	90	20	n/a	1	0	80	95	n/a	n/a	n/a	10
Ocean Perch, baked	100	20	0	2	0	50	80	*	*	10	6
Orange Roughy, broiled	70	16	0	1	0	20	70	*	*	*	*
Oyster, steamed, 12 medium	120	12	7	4	1	90	190	*	*	8	65
Pollack, broiled	100	21	0	1	0	80	90	*	*	*	*
Rainbow Trout, broiled	130	22	0	4	1	60	30	*	*	7	10
Rockfish, baked	100	20	0	2	0	40	65	4	*	*	3
Salmon, Atlantic/ Coho, baked	150	22	0	5	0	50	50	*	2	*	4
Shark, baked	140	22	n/a	5	1	50	80	n/a	n/a	n/a	5
Scallop, broiled, 6 large or 14 small	150	29	2	1	0	60	275	*	3	2	*
Shrimp, boiled	110	22	0	2	0	160	155	*	3	3	15
Sole, broiled	100	21	0	1	0	60	90	*	*	2	2
Swordfish, broiled	130	21	0	4	1	40	110	4	*	*	5
Tuna, Yellowfin, broiled	120	25	0	1	0	50	40	n/a	n/a	n/a	4
Whiting, baked	100	19	0	1	0	70	75	2	*	5	2

Serving Size: 3-ounce cooked portion—skinless, broiled/grilled, baked, microwaved, boiled, or steamed without additional fat, sodium, or sauces.
*Contains less than 2% of U.S. RDA.

Source: Nutritional Labeling Data provided by the Food and Drug Administration and Food Processor II™.

Defrosting Frozen Fish

Place the package of frozen fish in a dish and allow it to thaw for 24 hours in the refrigerator. Fish can be thawed in its original package under cold, running water, but this method will result in a loss of flavor and texture.

Cooking Tips

Fish should be cooked according to the "10 minutes per inch" rule, based on the maximum thickness of the fish. Steaks and thicker fillets should be turned halfway through the cooking time. Pieces of fish less than ½-inch thick do not have to be turned. Fillets should be placed skin side down. The skin will remove easily after cooking. If fillets are rolled or stuffed, measure at the thickest point to determine cooking time. Fish is done when the flesh begins to change from translucent to opaque or white and is firm but still moist. It should flake easily with a fork.

GRILLING

Place steaks or fillets on an oiled grill over medium-hot coals. Cover and cook without turning, or if left uncovered, turn halfway through cooking time. If using a stovetop grill, fill the basin with water and brush the surface of the grill lightly with oil. Cook over medium-high heat and provide adequate ventilation.

BROILING

Place steaks or fillets in a broiling pan and brush with marinade. Broil 3 to 6 inches from heat, basting frequently and turning steaks halfway through cooking.

POACHING

Simmer fillets or steaks in a stock, using a pan with a lid to retain heat. Turning is not necessary. Baste occasionally by spooning stock over fish.

PAN SAUTÉING

Heat a small amount of marinade or oil in a heavy skillet. For steaks or fillets over ½-inch thick, turn halfway through cooking time.

BAKING

Preheat oven to 450°F. Bake uncovered, basting if desired.

POULTRY

Poultry is a broad classification that covers the various species of domesticated and game birds. These include turkey, chicken, duck, goose, and wild birds. When cooking poultry, take the same precautions as when cooking meat or fish. Always make sure that the flesh is fully cooked before eating. If you see a pink tinge, even next to the bone, cook the poultry a little longer.

MILK AND CHEESES

The milk group includes milk, cheese, ice cream, yogurt, and kefir. The importance of milk in the diet has long been recognized. Calcium and phosphorus levels in milk are very high. Vitamin A levels are high in whole milk, but in the production of skim milk, this fat-soluble vitamin is removed. Riboflavin is present in significant quantities in milk unless the milk has been exposed to light. Though milk contains important amounts of most nutrients, it is very low in iron and ascorbic acid, and it is low in niacin. The composition of whole milk is approximately 4.9 percent carbohydrate, 3.5 percent fat, 3.5 percent protein, and about 87 percent water. The main carbohydrate in milk is lactose, or milk sugar. The most abundant fatty acids in milk are oleic, palmitic, and stearic acids. Milk is a complete protein food containing several protein complexes. The chief protein fraction in cow's milk is casein. The whey protein complex includes lactalbumin, lactoglobulin, and lactomucin.

Cheese is one of the oldest and most nutritious food products. It is formed by the coagulation of milk by rennet (the digestive enzyme in the stomach of the calf) or similar enzymes, and the draining off of the liquid whey. Part of the moisture is removed from the curd by cutting, warming, or pressing. Then it is usually shaped in a mold and ripened by storing for some time at a particular temperature and humidity. The ripening, or curing, process is the result of bacteriological processes. Processed cheese is a mixture of ground cheese (usually cheddar and other hard varieties), emulsifying salts such as phosphates, other ingredients such as milk powder, whey powder, and coloring and flavoring materials, and, sometimes, spices. Vegetable gum is often added to produce a chewy texture. Steam is blown into the mixture to raise the temperature to 150°F or higher, which yields a molten plasticlike mass that is then poured into a metal or ceramic container, or into portion-containers for foil wrapping.

Hard cheese, such as cheddar, is one of the most concentrated of common foods: 100 grams (about 3.5 oz.) supplies about 36 percent of the protein, 80 percent of the calcium, and 34 percent of the fat in the recommended daily allowance. Cheese is also a good source of some vitamins and minerals.

Nutritionally, milk is best preserved by condensing or drying, as none of the nutrients are lost. Conversion to cheese also is an excellent way to preserve the nutrients of milk, because virtually all the fat and most of the protein are retained, and the latter is partially digested. However, nearly all the sugar (lactose) and some of the minerals, protein, and vitamins escape into the whey. Because cheese is a high-protein food, it is an ideal nutritional replacement for meat in a vegetarian diet. It is rich in the essential amino acids, calcium, phosphorus, other minerals and vitamins, and it has a high caloric value.

One of the primary habits you will want to develop regarding cheeses is to read the labels. Cheeses vary so greatly in fat and calorie content that you will either want to see the breakdown on the label or learn about various full cut, unlabeled products yourself. In this way, you can become a savvy cheese eater.

Current Research

Nutrition research is ongoing and proliferating. Increasing evidence links food intake with both health and illness.

DAIRY FOODS AND BONE HEALTH

It is unclear whether dairy foods promote bone health in all populations and whether all dairy foods are equally beneficial. One review of scientific evidence supports the recommendation that dairy foods be consumed daily for improved bone health in the general U.S. population. Studies were reviewed that examined the relation of dairy foods to bone health in all age, sex, and race groups. Outcomes were classified according to the strength of the evidence by using a priori guidelines and were categorized as favorable, unfavorable, or not statistically significant. Of 57 outcomes of the effects of dairy foods on bone health, 53 percent were not significant, 42 percent were favorable, and 5 percent were unfavorable. Of 21 stronger evidence studies, 57 percent were not significant, 29 percent were favorable, and 14 percent were unfavorable. Dairy foods varied widely in their content of nutrients known to affect calcium excretion and skeletal mass. Foods such as milk and yogurt are likely to be beneficial; others, such as cottage cheese, may adversely affect bone health. Of the few stronger evidence studies of dairy foods and bone health, most had outcomes that were not significant. However, white women younger than 30 years are most likely to benefit. There are too few studies in males and minority ethnic groups to determine whether dairy foods promote bone health in most of the U.S. population (Weinsier & Krumdieck, 2000).

YOGURT CONSUMPTION AND IMMUNE FUNCTION

Fermented milk products may protect against breast cancer by stimulating immunologic activity. Twenty-five women were assigned randomly to two groups: control and yogurt treatment. Controls refrained from yogurt products for 3 months, while the yogurt treatment group consumed two cups of commercially produced yogurt for three consecutive months. Prior yogurt consumption did not exceed 4 to 6 cups per month, and subjects consumed their usual diet during the study. Three-day diet records and fasting midluteal blood samples were obtained during subjects' first, second, and fourth menstrual cycles (baseline, Month 1, and Month 3, respectively). Macronutrient intakes differed between groups only for carbohydrate. Calcium intake increased for yogurt consumers during intervention. Lymphocyte proliferation induced by concanavalin A, phytohemagglutinin, and pokeweed mitogen, interleukin 2 production, and cytotoxic T lymphocyte-mediated cytotoxicity was assessed after baseline and Months 1 and 3 for both groups. No significant immune differences between the control and yogurt treatment group were observed. In conclusion, three months of yogurt consumption did not enhance ex vivo cell-mediated immune function in young women (Campbell, Chew, Luedecke, & Shultz, 2000).

SUMMARY

Proteins are the most important part of nutrition. The human body is made of proteins and they play an essential role in how it functions. When dieting, when eating for energy, while exercising, during pregnancy, or in old age, protein needs must be met.

REFERENCES

Campbell, C. G., Chew, B. P., Luedecke, L. O., & Shultz, T. D. (2000). Yogurt consumption does not enhance immune function in healthy premenopausal women. *Nutrition and Cancer, 37*(1), 27–35.

Futterman, L. G., & Lemberg, L. (2001). Lp(a) lipoprotein—An independent risk factor for coronary heart disease after menopause. *American Journal of Critical Care, 10*(1), 63–67.

Ordovas, J. M. (2000). Genetic polymorphisms and activity of cholesterol ester transfer protein (CETP): Should we be measuring them? *Clinical Chemistry and Laboratory Medicine, 38*(10), 945–949.

Weinsier, R. L., & Krumdieck, C. L. (2000). Dairy foods and bone health: Examination of the evidence. *American Journal of Clinical Nutrition, 72*(3), 681–689.

Williams, J. A., Martin, F. L., Muir, G. H., Hewer, A., Grover, P. L., & Phillips, D. H. (2000). Metabolic activation of carcinogens and expression of various cytochromes P450 in human prostate tissue. *Carcinogenesis, 21*(9), 1683–1689.

CHAPTER 6

Fats

A generation ago we didn't know that smearing butter on sandwiches, deep fat frying, and eating red meat three times a day could be detrimental to our health. I remember my mother saving the morning bacon fat in a peanut butter jar that sat on the windowsill. It was added for flavoring to most meals and the daily fried eggs were splattered with it to cook the sunny tops. Beans were cooked with ham or bacon, and rich, full-fat butter coated everything. And, of course, the delicious country Sunday chicken was fried in lard.

These days we know a lot more and are consequently in the midst of a major dietary transition. Today, we have differentiated between hydrogenated and saturated fats and we know the difference between polysaturated and monosaturated fats. Each of these fats is different and some are better for us than others.

OVERVIEW

Lipids, which make up most of the rest of the body's weight (15 percent), serve as stores of food energy in the form of fat. More complex lipids, such as phospholipids, are basic constituents of cell membranes and steroids, which include hormones that perform other vital chemical functions. The following terms describe aspects of fat that we hear about frequently, but may need to brush up on for better understanding.

Saturated Fats

Saturated fats contain large numbers of hydrogen atoms in their chemical composition. They are suspected of raising blood cholesterol levels. Most saturated fats come from animal products. *Tropical* vegetable oils (palm kernel, palm, and coconut, particularly) are the only vegetable fats that are high in saturated fats. Saturated fats have been linked to an increased risk of coronary heart disease. A higher percentage of saturated fats can increase total blood cholesterol, especially the "bad" low-density lipoproteins (LDLs). Oils and fats with a high proportion of saturated fats include palm oil, coconut oil, and lard.

Hydrogenated Fats or Trans-Fatty Acids

Hydrogenated fats have undergone a process whereby hydrogen is bubbled through a polyunsaturated fat in order to give the otherwise liquid fat a harder consistency and more stability against rancidity. An example of a hydrogenated fat is margarine. Hydrogenated fats are no more healthy than comparable animal-based saturated fats. There are also concerns as to how the chemical nature of the fat is changed during hydrogenation and how usable these hydrogenated fats are in the body.

Polyunsaturated Fats

Polyunsaturated fats are considered physiologically less threatening and tend to decrease total blood cholesterol. Unfortunately, they also lower the amount of "good" blood cholesterol, or high-density lipoproteins (HDLs). Too many polyunsaturated fats in the diet may also increase the risk of some types of cancer. Linoleic acid (a polyunsaturated fat) has been found to enhance the growth of breast, pancreatic, and possibly colon cancer in rats. Oils and fats with a high proportion of polyunsaturated fats include soybean oil, corn oil, sunflower oil, safflower oil, and cottonseed oil. Vegetable oils (corn, cottonseed, soybean, safflower) contain large percentages of the polyunsaturated fatty acid linolenic acid. Peanut and sesame oils are fairly high in linolenic acid.

Monounsaturated Fats

Monounsaturated fats seem to help reduce levels of LDLs while preserving the beneficial HDLs. Oils high in monounsaturated fats include canola oil, olive oil, high-oleic safflower oil, peanut oil, and sesame oil. Studies show that in cultures where people use olive oil as the predominant fat, there tends to be a lower incidence of heart disease. An added advantage of monounsaturated fats is their naturally high resistance to rancidity. Because monounsaturated fats are basically healthy, and we do need fats in our diets, some facts about olive oil follow.

OLIVE OIL

Olive oil is one of the few oils in the world pressed from a fruit. It has been savored by Greeks and southern Italians for centuries, and these populations have surprisingly low rates of cardiovascular disease even with fairly high consumption of this fat. Olive oil is available in the following types:

Extra-virgin—the top grade, most expensive of the oils; naturally contains less than 1 percent acid. It is the most flavorful, with a fruity or peppery olive taste.

Virgin—contains 1 percent to 3.3 percent acid.

Refined—the lowest and least expensive grade; contains more than 3.3 percent acid.

Pure—a blend of virgin or extra-virgin with refined olive oil; contains no more than 3.3 percent acid.

Some information on the background of olive oils: where they grow, how they are harvested, and so on, follows.

- *Geographic and seasonal facts.* Soil, climate, and particular weather conditions all affect the characteristics of agricultural products such as grapes, milk, and olives. That is why only specific regions of the world, such as the Middle East and Mediterranean countries, cultivate olive trees.

- *Time of harvest.* The flavor of olives differs greatly from one plant to another. Flavor is due partly to the ripeness of the olive. Green olives picked in September or October have a sharper, fruitier flavor and a greener color than the darker, riper olives picked in November and December, which are sweeter and more subtle.

- *Method of harvest.* The best olive oils are made from hand-picked olives. Hand-picked olives do not get bruised and can be selected for the desired ripeness. These olives are made into the virgin or extra-virgin oils. Lower-quality oils are made from olives that have been mechanically harvested or have fallen to the ground.

- *Olive oil production.* The very best oils are from olives that are "cold-pressed" between mill stones after drying for 2 to 3 days to reduce the water content. Traditional small olive oil producers run their mills continuously so the olives can be pressed at their peak condition.

- *Storage of olive oil.* Store olive oil in a cool, dark place, making sure it is not exposed to direct light. In hot climates, it can be stored in the refrigerator, but unrefined extra-virgin oil will solidify. It will melt back into a liquid upon standing at room temperature. It is best to use a bottle or tin of olive oil within a year of purchase.

- *Uses for olive oil.* Olive oil is excellent when combined with vinegar for salad dressings, tossed with pasta, used as a sauté base for stovetop meals, or substituted for butter or margarine on bread.

- *Caloric content.* Like all oils, olive oil contains 120 calories and 14 grams of fat per tablespoon. Consequently, no matter how good a replacement it is for other kinds of fat, it should be used with discretion.

CHOLESTEROL

Cholesterol is a waxy substance made primarily in the liver and in the cells lining the small intestine. It is an essential constituent of cell membranes and nerve fibers, and is a building block of certain hormones. It is found in all body tissues, but the cholesterol that circulates in the blood creates the most concern. Fats (triglycerides) and cholesterol are transported through the bloodstream in protein-wrapped clusters called lipoproteins, which are assembled in the liver and intestinal tract. These lipoproteins are labeled according to their density, based on the proportion of triglycerides, phospholipids, cholesterol, and protein they contain.

Total Cholesterol

Total cholesterol reflects the total amount of artery-clogging cholesterol in the blood. The National Cholesterol Education Program designates blood levels less than 200 mg/dl as desirable; levels between 200 and 240 mg/dl as borderline-high; and those over 240 mg/dl as indicative of a greater risk of heart disease. The three other lipid values are measurements of lipoproteins, the special proteins that carry cholesterol through the vascular system.

VERY LOW DENSITY LIPOPROTEINS (VLDL)

VLDLs contain 55 to 65 percent triglycerides, 5 to 10 percent protein, 10 to 15 percent cholesterol, and 15 to 20 percent phospholipids. Their job is to carry triglycerides to the cells for use or to other parts of the body for storage. After the VLDLs deposit their triglycerides and undergo other changes, they become low density lipoproteins.

LOW DENSITY LIPOPROTEINS (LDL)

LDLs contain 45 percent cholesterol, 25 percent moderate protein, 10 percent triglycerides, and 22 percent phospholipids. These lipoproteins have become known as *bad* cholesterol because after they deliver the cholesterol actually needed by the cells, they deposit any excess in arterial walls and other tissues.

HIGH DENSITY LIPOPROTEINS (HDL)

HDLs contain the highest amount of protein (45 to 50 percent), 5 percent triglycerides, 20 percent cholesterol, and 30 percent phospholipids. HDL lipoproteins pick up the cholesterol deposits and bring them to the liver for recycling or disposal; thus they are known as the *good* cholesterol. A higher proportion of HDL to LDLs represents more active cholesterol, a lowered risk of developing atherosclerosis, and a lower risk of heart attack and stroke.

Sensitivity to Dietary Cholesterol

The molecular mechanisms regulating the amount of dietary cholesterol retained in the body, as well as the body's ability to exclude selectively other dietary sterols, are poorly understood. An average Western diet contains about 250 to 500 mg of dietary cholesterol and about 200 to 400 mg of noncholesterol sterols. About 50 percent to 60 percent of the dietary cholesterol is absorbed and retained by the normal human body, but less than 1 percent of the noncholesterol sterols are retained. Thus, there exists a subtle mechanism that allows the body to distinguish between cholesterol and noncholesterol sterols (Lee et al., 2001).

It is theorized that 20 to 30 percent of the U.S. population are genetically hypersensitive to dietary cholesterol and, therefore, have blood cholesterol levels that increase when they eat high-cholesterol foods. Since there is no simple test for cholesterol hypersensitivity, it is suggested that everyone monitor their intake of dietary cholesterol.

Cholesterol is found only in foods of animal origin: meat, eggs, poultry, fish, and dairy products, including butter. Fruits, vegetables, grains, and legumes contain no cholesterol. Saturated fats in foods usually stimulate the production of LDL (bad) cholesterol and raise overall cholesterol levels. Therefore, even if a low-cholesterol diet is maintained, a diet high in saturated fats can still mean trouble.

New understanding of the important role of HDLs in protecting against heart disease led a National Institutes of Health panel to recommend that all adults know their HDL and total cholesterol levels. Bringing abnormal lipid levels within normal parameters lowers the risk factors for heart disease. For every 1 percent drop in total cholesterol, the risk of heart disease declines 2 to 3 percent; and every 1 mg/dl higher increment in HDL reduces heart disease by another 2 to 3 percent.

Taking cholesterol-lowering drugs can reduce levels. A low-fat diet lowers cholesterol about 10 percent, whereas adding cholesterol-lowering drugs to a low-fat diet can bring a 20 percent reduction. The decision to supplement a low-fat diet with pharmaceutical aids depends on an individual's complete risk profile: total cholesterol and lipoprotein levels, family history, prior myocardial infarction or stroke, smoking, obesity, and hypertension.

RISK FACTORS

Risk factors are based on determination of high, moderate, or low risk for heart disease. Risk factors are determined by evaluating the person's current cholesterol level, weight, prior family history, smoking history, exercise patterns, and intake of high cholesterol and highly saturated foods. The following recommendations of the American Heart Association are based on risk group category.

High. Eat no more than 20 percent of your total calories from fat, and reduce cholesterol to 100–150 mg per day.

Moderate. Eat no more than 25 percent of your total calories from fat, and reduce cholesterol to 200–250 mg per day.

Low. Eat no more than 30 percent of your total calories from fat, and reduce cholesterol to 200–300 mg per day.

Fats are usually calculated or measured in grams of fat. Table 6–1 (on pages 78–79) lists the number of grams of fat for most of the common foods. The following list explains ways to reduce fat consumption.

- *Know your numbers.* Total cholesterol should be less than 200mg/dl. Levels over 240 mg/dl demand attention. HDL cholesterol should be over 35 mg/dl. Less than 35 mg/dl demands attention. Above 45 mg/dl is even better. LDL cholesterol should be less than 160 mg/dl. The ratio of total cholesterol to HDL cholesterol is best if below 4.5; above 5.5 is undesirable. Lipoprotein should be less than 0.3 g/l.

- *Get a lipid analysis.* Do not rely on a simple cholesterol test. Research indicates that abnormal levels of lipids can be corrected when we know our levels and are motivated to change.

- *Follow dietary restrictions prior to the test.* A 12-hour fast is necessary for an accurate measurement of LDL cholesterol and triglycerides.

- *Have a follow-up lipid test every five years, if the results are normal.* If one or more values fall outside the desirable range, get more frequent tests.

- *Make necessary lifestyle changes.* A low-fat, low-cholesterol diet will help bring lipid abnormalities in line. Maintaining optimum weight and regular exercise can boost HDL levels.

- *Eliminate other risk factors.* If you smoke, stop. If you are overweight, reduce. If you are sedentary, begin to move. Seek medical attention for diabetes, hypertension, or when there is a family history of dietary-related problems.

HOW MUCH FAT DO WE NEED?

Most nutritionists concur that we need to limit all fats to 30 percent of our total caloric intake. Of that amount, saturated fats should constitute less than 10 percent of our total daily requirements. The remaining 20 percent should be divided between polyunsaturated and monounsaturated fats. This means that for a diet of approximately 2,000 calories per day, 600 of the calories may come from fats. The American Heart Association recommends more specific guidelines and suggests that fewer than 10 percent of daily calories come from saturated fats and fewer than 10 percent come from polyunsaturated fats. Monounsaturated fats should make up the rest. Because a tablespoon of oil contains about 120 calories, we can consume up to 5 tablespoons of oil and still remain within the 30 percent guideline if our calorie needs are around 2,000 calories per day. However, these 5 tablespoons also include all the hidden fats found in baked goods, candy, meats, fish, poultry, nuts, seeds, peanut butter, eggs, and salad dressings, as well as the oil and butter we use to sauté or flavor foods. If we take in 2,000 calories a day, that means consuming fewer than 67 grams of fat (1 gram of fat provides 9 calories, so 67 grams x 9 calories/gram = 603 calories). If we consume 1,500 calories a day we need to keep daily fat intake under 50 grams.

What Is the Difference Between Margarine and Butter?

BUTTER

Butter is a delicately flavored dairy food made from milk fat to which salt and coloring are usually added. It is believed that the saturated fatty acids found in butter, milk, and other animal products can raise the level of cholesterol in the blood, thus leading to arteriosclerosis.

MARGARINE

Margarine is a hydrogenated fat similar to the hardened vegetable shortenings sold in cans. The hydrogenation process involves adding hydrogen atoms to soybean, corn, and other liquid oils to make the oils more solid and resistant to rancidity. This process changes many of the unsaturated fatty acids, making them more saturated and transforming their chemical structures. Appropriately, these altered fats are called *trans-fatty acids*. The more solid the margarine, the more trans-fatty acids it contains. Consequently, stick margarines contain more trans-fatty acids than tub brands, and tubs have more than the squeeze-bottle products. Concerns are that trans-fatty acids may increase the risk of heart disease, cancer, and possibly other problems. Margarine has been found to contain transmonounsaturated fatty acids which form during the processing. These fatty acids raise cholesterol levels.

TABLE 6-1 Grams of Fat for Common Foods

Meats—Poultry (1 oz. cooked)

Food	Grams
Chicken, broilers or fryers, dark meat with skin, roasted	4
Chicken, dark meat without skin, roasted	3
Chicken, light meat with skin, roasted	3
Chicken, light meat without skin, roasted	1
Chicken frankfurter, about 2	6
Turkey bacon	10
Turkey bologna, about 3½ slices	4
Turkey frankfurter, about 2	5
Turkey, light meat with skin, roasted	3
Turkey, light meat without skin, roasted	1

Meats—Beef (1 oz. cooked)

Food	Grams
Bologna, cured, 3–4 slices	8
Chuck, arm pot roast, lean only, braised	3
Ground, lean, broiled, medium	5
Hot dog, cured, about 2	8
Hot dog, 97% fat free	0.5
Hot dog, 90% fat free	3
Round, bottom round, lean only, braised	3
Round, top round, lean only, broiled	2
Sausage, cured, cooked, smoked, about 2	8

Meats—Pork (1 oz. cooked)

Food	Grams
Bacon, Canadian	1
Breakfast strips	7
Bacon, fried	14
Cured ham, boneless, regular, roasted	3
Cured, smoked link sausage, grilled	9
Fresh, loin, center loin, lean and fat, roasted	6
Fresh, loin, tenderloin, lean only, roasted	1

Meats—Fish and Shellfish (1 oz. cooked)

Food	Grams
Haddock, dry heat	0.3
Salmon, sockeye, dry heat	3
Tuna, bluefin, dry heat	2
Lobster, northern	0.2
Oyster, Eastern, moist heat	1
Shrimp, mixed species	0.3

Dairy and Egg Products

Food	Grams
American processed cheese food, 1 oz.	7
Cheddar, 1 oz.	9
Cottage cheese, creamed, 4 oz.	5
Cottage cheese, 1% fat, 4 oz.	1
Cream cheese, 1 oz.	10
Mozzarella, 1 oz.	6
Mozzarella, part skim, 1 oz.	5
Muenster, 1 oz.	9
Parmesan, 1 oz.	9
Provolone, 1 oz.	8
Ricotta, part skim, 4 oz.	9
Ricotta, whole milk, 4 oz.	15
Swiss, 1 oz.	8

Eggs

Food	Grams
Egg, chicken, white	trace (tr)
Egg, chicken, whole	6

Frozen Desserts

Food	Grams
Frozen yogurt, fruit-flavored, low-fat	2
Fudgesicle	0.2
Frozen yogurt, nonfat	0
Frozen yogurt, regular	7
Ice cream, vanilla, regular	14
Ice milk, vanilla, soft serve	5
Pudding pops, 1 pop	3
Sherbet, orange	4

Milk (8 oz.)

Food	Grams
Buttermilk	2
Chocolate shake	11
Low-fat milk, 1% fat	3
Low-fat milk, 2% fat	5
Skim milk	0.4
Whole milk, 3.3% fat	8

Yogurt (4 oz.)

Food	Grams
Plain yogurt	4
Plain yogurt, low-fat	0.2

Nuts and Seeds (1 oz.)

Item	Grams
Almonds	15
Cashew nuts	13
Peanuts	14
Pecans	18

Breads, Cereals, Pasta, Rice, and Dried Peas and Beans

Item	Grams
Biscuits, buttermilk or oven-ready, 3"	3
Croissant, 4½"	12
Doughnut, 3¼"	12
Danish	8
French bread, 1–2 oz.	1
Muffin, 2½"	5–6
Pancake, 4"	2
Raisin, biscuit	7
Rolls, brown & serve, 1 each	2
Rolls, crescent, 1 each	4–6
Rolls, dinner, butterflake, 1 each	5
Waffle, 7"	13
Waffle, lite	2
Wheat/white bread, 2 slices	1
Turnover, cherry	19
Granola type (¼ cup)	6

Pasta (1 cup)

Item	Grams
Chow mein noodles	11
Egg noodles, cooked	2

Sweets and Snacks

Cakes and Pies

Item	Grams
Apple pie, ⅛ of 9" pie	13
Cream pie, ⅛ of 9" pie	17
Gingerbread, ⅛ of 8" cake	4
Layer cake with icing, ⅛ of 9" cake	8–9
Lemon meringue pie, ⅛ of 9" pie	11
Pound cake, 1/17 of loaf	5
Pudding, ½ cup	4

Candy

Item	Grams
Banana chips, ¼ cup	12
Butterfingers/Nestle Crunch, ¼ cup	6
Chocolate chips, ¼ cup	12
Fudge, 1 oz.	3
Gummi bears, ¼ cup	0
Jelly beans, ¼ cup	0

Sweets and Snacks (cont.)

Candy

Item	Grams
M&M (peanut), ¼ cup	14
M&M (plain), 1 oz.	9
Milk chocolate, plain, ¼ cup	13
Raisinettes, ¼ cup	8
Reese's Pieces, ¼ cup	10
Yogurt-covered raisins, ¼ cup	16

Snacks

Item	Grams
Corn chips, 1 oz.	9
Popcorn, with oil, 1 cup	3
Popcorn, air popped, 1 cup	tr
Potato chips, 1 oz.	10
Pretzels, stick, 2¼", 10 pretzels	tr

Miscellaneous

Item	Grams
Pizza, cheese ⅛ of 15" diameter	9

Fats and Oils

Item	Grams
Margarine, diet, 1 tsp.	2
Margarine, liquid, bottled, 1 tsp.	3
Margarine, soft, tub, 1 tsp.	2
Margarine, stick, 1 tsp.	4

Salad Dressing (1 Tbsp.)

Item	Grams
Bleu cheese	8
French	6
Imitation mayonnaise	3
Italian	7
Low-calorie	1–2
Mayonnaise	11
Ranch	6
Thousand Island	6

Other

Item	Grams
Avocado, Florida	27
Gravies, canned, ½ cup	3–7
Nondairy creamer, powdered, 1 tsp.	1
Olives, green, 4 medium	1.5
Peanut butter, 1 tbsp.	7
Sour cream, 2 tbsp.	5

Recent reports indicate that diets high in trans-fatty acids raise the bad LDL cholesterol almost as much as saturated fats. More significant is that, unlike the other diets, the trans-fatty diet also lowers the good HDL cholesterol, suggesting that it may increase coronary risk as much as the high saturated-fat diet.

Since margarine and butter both can cause problems, choosing one over the other can be difficult. Minimizing both and alternating which one you use could be a way of improving your odds. For other ideas, read on.

Alternatives to Butter and Margarine

If both butter and margarine are dubious for good health, then what can we use for flavoring and cooking? Probably the best place to start is to reduce all fats in general and minimize foods high in saturated fats. If you choose to use margarine, try liquid or "squeeze" margarines instead of the more hydrogenated stick versions. The first ingredient listed on the label should be a liquid rather than a partially hydrogenated oil and the product should contain twice as much unsaturated fat as saturated. Avoid any brands with preservatives and artificial color.

The best alternative may be to substitute natural monounsaturated oils. Liquid vegetable oils (olive, canola, or peanut) can be used in cooking and baking. Bite-size pieces of fresh breads can be dipped into a small saucer of olive oil.

BASIC DIETARY CHANGES TO REDUCE FAT

The easiest way to maintain a low-fat, low-cholesterol meal plan is to use low-fat products and to prepare foods with minimal fat additives. Begin your dietary lifestyle change by choosing one, two, or three of the following practices and gradually include the others.

- Broil, bake, or steam instead of frying foods in fat.
- Use skim milk or low-fat milk and milk products.
- Limit intake of meats, fish, and poultry to 5 to 6 ounces per day and trim the fat.
- Substitute meatless or low-meat main dishes for regular entrées (see Chapter 14 on vegetarianism).
- Limit use of shrimp, lobster, sardines, and organ meats.
- Eat fatty fish once or twice weekly. They contain Omega-3 fatty acids, which lower blood cholesterol and triglycerides.
- Avoid foods containing hydrogenated vegetable shortenings, lard, hydrogenated or partially hydrogenated vegetable oils, coconut oil, palm kernel oil, and palm oil.

- Use vegetable oils in cooking. Use no more than a total of 5 to 8 teaspoons of fats and oils per day for cooking, baking, and salads.
- Use no more than three egg yolks per week.

Try using egg whites or cholesterol-free frozen egg products in cooking or baking. In baking, one whole egg equals two egg whites plus 1 teaspoon of oil. Many recipes work with two egg whites substituted for one whole egg.

RESEARCH STUDIES

An impressive body of evidence strongly supports the concept that multiple dietary factors influence blood pressure and that modification of diet can have powerful, beneficial effects on this highly prevalent cardiovascular risk factor. Dietary therapies proven to lower blood pressure include reduced sodium intake, weight loss, moderation of alcohol intake, increased potassium intake, and a diet that is low in fat and cholesterol, and that emphasizes fruits, vegetables, and low-fat dairy products. Several other dietary factors, such as an increased intake of protein or monounsaturated fatty acids, may also reduce blood pressure, but evidence to date is insufficient for policy recommendations. Still, widespread implementation of those therapies with a proven ability to lower blood pressure should have an enormous impact on the adverse patterns of blood pressure that remain highly prevalent in the United States and most other countries (Appel, 2000).

Current Research on Cholesterol-Lowering Diets

Increasing numbers of studies document the role of excess cholesterol and the development of cardiovascular and other diseases. One study assessed the impact of culturally sensitive modifications to the Duke University Rice Diet weight loss program for African American dieters. The study was a randomized modified crossover study in which volunteers received either early or delayed weight loss intervention. Final outcomes were measured at 8 weeks. At the onset of the study, there were 56 African American participants; however, only 79 percent completed the study. The eight-week intervention was a modified 1,000-calorie/day version of the Rice Diet. Modifications to the program included decreased cost, culturally sensitive recipes, addressing attitudes about exercise, and including family members in weight loss efforts. Average weight loss for subjects completing the program was 14.8 pounds. Body mass index (BMI) decreased from 37.8 kg/m2 to 35.3 kg/m2. Total cholesterol levels decreased from 199.2 mg/dl to 185.4 mg/dl; systolic and diastolic blood pressure decreased by 4.3 mmHg and 2.4 mmHg, respectively. The control group showed no significant change in any outcome measures. These results tell us that programs can be successfully tailored to incorporate the needs of African Americans. Most important, these dietary program changes can lead to significant health improvements (Ard, Rosati, & Oddone, 2000).

In another study, three composite diet samples were obtained based on seven-day weighed food records representing the traditional Cretan Mediterranean diet (diet A), the typical diet of present-day Greek adolescents (diet B), and the fasting diet of the Eastern Orthodox church (diet C). Chemical analyses provided a definitive measure, for the first time, of the nutrient composition of the complete Greek diet as it was in the early 1960s. In comparing chemical analyses with nutrient database analyses, differences greater than 15 percent were found in all three diets for cholesterol and some vitamins. The differences in total fat and saturated fat content were less than 15 percent in all diets. This study provides two practical examples of the Mediterranean diet, which although widely publicized has rarely been analyzed chemically. Diet A has been shown to be related to the lowest rates for coronary heart disease and cancer mortality compared with the diets of the other populations of the Seven Countries study. As such, it could be recommended for health promotion and prevention of disease. Diet C contains even lower amounts of saturated fatty acids and would be excellent for patients with hypercholesterolemia. The high antioxidants in diet C probably maintain very low levels of low-density lipoprotein cholesterol (Kafatos, Verhagen, Moschandreas, Apostolaki, & Van Westerop, 2000).

Medication to Lower Cholesterol

Coronary heart disease remains a major therapeutic challenge in the Western world, and strategies aimed at lowering cholesterol form the mainstay of treatment. In addition to changing nutrition habits, or while in the midst of change, new studies indicate that fluvastatin, at therapeutic doses, does lower cholesterol (Corsini, 2000). In cases such as hypercholesteremia health care providers have the opportunity to offer both conventional and alternative choices.

SUMMARY

Fats play a complex part in our lives. Having too much, too little, or the wrong variety of this lipid can affect our health. The intake of too much fat and cholesterol often leads to some aspect of coronary heart disease (CHD). Because the main cause of death in patients with CHD is sudden cardiac death, health care providers will want to develop specific strategies, including dietary changes, to prevent it. In the long term, reduction of the diet-dependent chronic risk factors of CHD, hypercholesterolemia, and hypertension is very important. The association of the cardioprotective effects of the Mediterranean diet with those expected from the reduction of blood lipids and blood pressure renders this dietary pattern extremely attractive for public health purposes (de Lorgeril & Salen, 2000).

All of us will want to personally look for ways to reduce risk factors that we know. By following these guidelines, we will be in a better position to assist those in our care.

REFERENCES

Appel, L. J. (2000). The role of diet in the prevention and treatment of hypertension. *Current Atherosclerosis Reports, 2*(6), 521–528.

Ard, J. D., Rosati, R., & Oddone, E. Z. (2000). Culturally sensitive weight loss program produces significant reduction in weight, blood pressure, and cholesterol in eight weeks. *Journal of the National Medical Association, 92*(11), 515–523.

Corsini, A. (2000). Fluvastatin: Effects beyond cholesterol lowering. *Journal of Cardiovascular Pharmacology and Therapeutics, 5*(3), 161–175.

de Lorgeril, M., & Salen, P. (2000). Diet as preventive medicine in cardiology. *Current Opinions in Cardiology, 15*(5), 364–370.

Kafatos, A., Verhagen, H., Moschandreas, J., Apostolaki, I., & Van Westerop, J. J. (2000). Mediterranean diet of Crete: Foods and nutrient content. *Journal of the American Dietetic Association, 100*(12), 1487–1493.

Lee, M. H., Lu, K., Hazard, S., Yu, H., Shulenin, S., Hidaka, H., Kojima, H., Allikmets, R., Sakuma, N., Pegoraro, R., Srivastava, A. K., Salen, G., Dean, M., & Patel, S. B. (2001). Identification of a gene, ABCG5, important in the regulation of dietary cholesterol absorption. *Nature Genetics, 27*(1), 79–83.

Carbohydrates

Susie was an active operating room technician. She was a skilled professional, but had a problem in her personal life. The problem was that she was round, entirely too round for what she should be in her late twenties. True, she had two children, but it had been four years since the last baby was born. No matter how hard she tried, the pounds and flab prevailed. Susie, like many women, remained chubby after childbirth. She was embarrassed by her weight and wore large, loose-fitting clothes. She opted to wear scrubs and work in an out-of-the-way area in the hospital. She felt comfortable there, especially since many of her colleagues were plump too. How did Susie get this way? In this chapter, we will explore the world of carbohydrates and their role in healing nutrition. We will attempt to answer the question about Susie's weight. Carbohydrates are essential for good health, but like all other foods, they must be consumed in moderation.

OVERVIEW

Carbohydrates are the most abundant and least expensive food sources of energy. Important dietary carbohydrates are divided into two basic groups: starches and sugars. Starches, which may be converted into utilizable sugars in plants or in the human body, are supplied in grains, pulses, tubers, and some rhizomes and roots. Sugars occur in many plants and fruits. The most important food commodity among the sugars is sucrose, which is obtained from sugarcane or the sugar beet.

Carbohydrates, which include cellulose, starches, sugars, and many other compounds, are the most abundant single class of organic substances found in nature. They are formed in green plants and certain bacteria by photosynthesis, in which energy derived from sunlight is used for the assimilation of carbon dioxide from the air. If carbon dioxide, water, minerals, and an appropriate inorganic source of nitrogen are available, these organisms, with the aid of solar energy, can synthesize all the different carbohydrates, proteins, and lipids they need for their existence. Other organisms cannot do this. It follows that life on Earth ultimately depends on this process of carbon dioxide assimilation in which carbohydrates are the first intermediates.

In animal tissues, acid carbohydrates occur in the cell coats of cartilage, bone, and other tissues and form the ground substance between connective tissue cells. The cell walls of bacteria consist of a rigid framework of sugar-polymer chains linked to peptide chains. The glycoproteins, which contain covalently attached carbohydrate groups, are widely distributed in cell membranes. In red blood corpuscles, the carbohydrate side chains determine the blood group type.

Carbohydrates also serve as storage products of energy. The principal storage forms are starch in plants and glycogen in animal tissues. Glycogen consists of polymers, or chains of glucose, that are deposited in cells in the form of granules when a surplus of glucose is available. In times of metabolic need, the polymers are broken down by enzymatic action and become fuel.

Single units of carbohydrates known as monosaccharides, or simple sugars, are compounds with either an aldehyde group or a ketone group. Monosaccharides are classified as trioses, tetroses, pentoses, and so on, indicating the number of carbon atoms in a molecule.

The use of carbohydrates by oxidation occurs in a reaction that is the reverse of that of photosynthesis. In plants, glucose is stored as starch and sucrose. In humans, excess glucose is stored as glycogen and is also converted to fat and stored in adipose tissues. Carbohydrate metabolic processes such as these are subject to regulatory controls in which various hormones play a predominant role.

SUGAR

Carbohydrates include simple sugars and giant polymers of such sugars. Sugars serve as sources of cellular energy, as building blocks for certain complex molecules, and as a way to store energy in the form of glycogen. Sugars are a diverse and important subdivision of naturally occurring carbohydrates. They are generally sweet tasting, dissolve easily in water, and form white or clear crystals when purified. Common table sugar, or sucrose, is but one of many kinds of sugars. Sugars are rapidly digested and provide a quick source of energy. They play an important but often controversial role in the diet.

Types of Sugars

Monosaccharides—simple sugars that have three to seven carbon atoms, in either a chain or a ring structure. Glucose and fructose are representative monosaccharides. Glucose is the sugar into which all digested carbohydrates are metabolized in the body. The term *blood sugar* refers to glucose levels in the blood. A malfunctioning of glucose metabolism can result in hypoglycemia, or low blood sugar. Glucose is used commercially as a sweetener, especially in wines and drugs. Fructose is used both as a sweetener and as a food preservative. The simple sugars ribose and deoxyribose are major constituents of the nucleic acids RNA and DNA, respectively.

Disaccharides—consist of two simple sugars linked together. Maltose, for instance, is composed of two glucose molecules, and lactose consists of a glucose and a galactose molecule. Sucrose can be broken down into the simple sugars glucose and fructose.

Polysaccharides—large chains of simple sugars that form such polysaccharides as cellulose, glycogen, and starch.

Sugarcane and sugar beets—the principal commercial sources of sucrose. Maple sap, sorghum, and some palm and date trees also yield limited quantities of sucrose.

FRUITS AND VEGETABLES

Remember when you were a child? If you lived on a farm or in a family who grew gardens, summertime may remind you of the abundance of fresh fruits and vegetables. Plates heaped with fresh green beans and new red potatoes were common fare. Desserts were berry pies or cobblers and Sunday afternoons always included watermelons. Ripe, dripping, succulent tomatoes were available directly from the vine. The freshest of healthy fruits and vegetables were a part of everyday summer life. With careful shopping they still can be today.

Vegetables

Most vegetables are important sources of minerals, vitamins, and cellulose. Some vegetables, such as potatoes, corn, and peas, contribute appreciable quantities of starch and, in some people, may be the culprit in excess calorie intake. A ½-cup serving of these vegetables, which have visible, white starch in the center, is equivalent in calories to one slice of bread. Balancing your intake of starchy vegetables with plenty of low-calorie vitamin- and mineral-rich ones, such as carrots, broccoli, and spinach, is vital to a healthy diet.

Vegetables, particularly spinach, beans, and soybean products, contain large amounts of the minerals calcium and iron. Greens are high in calcium, while lentils and split peas are high in iron. Vegetables also help to meet the body's need for sodium, chloride, cobalt, copper, magnesium, manganese, phosphorus, and potassium. Carotenes (the precursor of vitamin A) and ascorbic acid (vitamin C) are abundant in many vegetables. Vegetables are useful in the diet for their cellulose content. Very little, if any, cellulose is digested in the body, but cellulose provides the roughage (fiber) required to promote motility of food through the intestines.

Fruits

One of the best things about fresh fruit is that it is filling without adding too many calories. For the same number of calories in a regular-sized candy bar, you could eat three apples, which contain virtually no fat. Citrus fruits are a valuable source of vitamin C, and yellow fruits, such as peaches, contain carotene. Dried fruits contain an ample amount of iron, although these fruits contain more calories in a smaller volume. Figs and oranges are excellent sources of calcium.

Like vegetables, fruits have a high cellulose content and provide fiber to protect against hemorrhoids, diverticulitis, and some forms of colon cancer. The fruit fiber pectin seems to lower blood cholesterol levels and evidence suggests that this fiber may help regulate blood pressure. Many fruits are rich in potassium, which is necessary for muscle contraction, maintenance of fluid and electrolyte balance in cells, transmission of nerve impulses, and energy release during metabolism.

To get the most nutritional value from fruit, buy it as ripe as possible and eat it within a few days. The nutrients begin to diminish after the fruits are picked. Table 7–1 details the nutritional benefits of the most popular fruits. Table 7–2 (on page 90) details nutrient information of the most available fruits.

GRAINS

Cereal grains are the least expensive source of calories for human consumption. An important energy source, they supply most of the carbohydrates in the human diet throughout the world. The proteins, lipids, vitamins, and minerals contained in cereals are also of considerable nutritional importance. The carbohydrate content of cereals ranges from 60 to 80 percent; lipid content ranges from 2 to 7 percent. The variability of the constituents is illustrated by the range of protein content within the grains: barley, 8 to 21 percent; corn, 8 to 17 percent; rye, 8 to 10 percent; wheat, 8 to 22 percent. The extent and method of processing drastically alter the vitamin, mineral, and lipid values.

Most grains are milled to separate the floury endosperm from the bran and germ, which can cause rancidity. The germ is nutritious, however, and is often added to food products after being dried and rolled. The oil extracted from the

TABLE 7–1	**Nutritional Benefits of Fresh Fruits**
FRUITS	**BENEFITS**
Apple	A good source of fiber
Apricot	Rich in beta-carotene; also contains potassium; a good source of fiber
Banana	High in potassium and vitamin B_6; a good source of fiber
Blackberry	Contains vitamin C; a good source of fiber
Cantaloupe	Rich in beta-carotene, vitamin C, thiamine, and potassium
Cherry	Contains potassium
Grapefruit	High in vitamin C
Grape	High in fiber
Honeydew melon	High in vitamin C, thiamine, and potassium
Kiwi fruit	Especially rich in vitamin C; good source of fiber
Mango	High in beta-carotene and vitamin C; good source of fiber
Nectarine	High in beta-carotene; contains vitamin E and potassium; good source of fiber
Orange	Especially rich in vitamin C; a good source of fiber
Papaya	High in vitamin C; also contains beta-carotene and potassium
Peach	High in beta-carotene; a good source of fiber
Pear	A good source of fiber; also contains potassium
Pineapple	High in potassium; contains vitamin C
Plum	A good source of vitamin A and fiber
Raspberry	High in niacin; also contains vitamin C; a good source of fiber
Strawberry	Especially rich in vitamin C; a good source of fiber
Watermelon	Rich in beta-carotene and potassium; contains vitamins B_6, C, and thiamine

germ is refined for salad or cooking use. Most processed by-products of grain are used as feed. Flour is used in various types of baked and cereal products, pasta products, and gravies. Pearled, rolled, flaked, ground, and cut grains are used in breakfast foods, soup, meal, hominy, and specialty items.

CARBOHYDRATE ADDICTION

Not all of us can eat carbohydrates with impunity. Some of us get a taste and then develop a craving. Some nutritionists believe that this craving is a carbohydrate addiction characterized by a compelling desire for high-carbohydrate foods such as candy, ice cream, pastries, cookies, sugary sodas, cakes, and pies. This disorder, known as hyperinsulinemia, strikes a lot of us, causing us to gain large amounts of

TABLE 7–2 Fruit Nutrition Information

FRUIT	Total Calories KCAL	Protein G	Carbohydrates G	Total Fat G	Dietary Fiber MG	Sodium MG	Vitamin A % U.S. RDA	Vitamin C % U.S. RDA	Calcium % U.S. RDA	Iron % U.S. RDA
Apple, 1 med.	80	0	18	1	5	0	*	6	*	*
Apricot, 2 med.	35	1	8	0	1	1	18	12	*	2
Avocado, ⅓ med.	120	1	2	12	2	5	*	5	*	*
Banana, 1 med.	120	1	28	1	3	0	*	15	*	*
Blackberry, 1 cup	75	1	18	1	10	0	2	50	5	5
Blueberry, 1 cup	80	1	21	1	4	9	*	32	*	2
Cantaloupe, 1 cup cubed	45	1	11	0	1	12	43	93	2	2
Carambala (starfruit), 1 med.	40	1	10	0	2	3	6	50	*	2
Casaba melon, 1 cup cubed	45	1	11	0	2	20	*	45	*	4
Cherry, 1 cup	90	1	19	1	3	0	*	10	2	*
Coconut, 1″ x 1.5″ piece	80	1	3	8	2	5	*	2	*	3
Cranberry, 1 cup	50	0	12	0	4	1	*	15	*	*
Figs, 2 med.	75	1	19	0	4	7	*	3	4	2
Grapes, 1.5 cups	85	1	24	0	2	3	3	9	2	2
Grapefruit, ½ med.	50	1	14	0	6	0	6	90	4	*
Honeydew melon, 1 cup cubed	60	1	16	0	2	17	*	70	*	*
Kiwi, 2 med.	90	1	18	1	4	0	2	230	4	4
Kumquat, 6 med.	70	1	19	0	4	7	3	72	5	2
Loquat, 10 med.	50	0	12	0	0	1	15	2	*	2
Lemon, 1 med.	18	0	4	0	0	10	*	35	2	*
Lime, 1 med.	20	0	7	0	3	1	*	35	2	2
Mango, ½ med.	65	1	18	0	4	2	40	48	*	*
Nectarine, 1 med.	70	1	16	1	3	0	20	10	*	*
Orange, 1 med.	50	1	13	0	6	0	*	120	4	*
Papaya, ½ med.	60	1	15	0	3	5	4	27	*	5
Passion fruit, 3 small	55	1	13	0	9	15	4	27	*	5
Peach, 2 med.	70	1	19	0	1	0	20	20	*	*
Pear, 1 med.	100	1	25	1	4	1	*	10	2	2
Persimmon, ½ large	60	0	16	0	2	1	18	10	*	*
Pineapple, ½″ slice	90	1	21	1	2	10	*	35	*	*
Plantain, ½ med	80	1	21	0	3	3	7	20	*	2
Plum, 2 med.	70	1	17	1	1	0	9	20	*	*
Pomegranate, ½ med.	50	1	13	0	1	2	*	8	*	*
Prickly pear, 1 med.	40	1	10	1	2	5	*	23	6	2
Raspberry, 1 cup	60	1	14	1	8	0	*	52	2	4
Strawberry, 8 med.	50	1	13	0	30	0	*	140	2	2
Tamarind, 1 med.	5	0	1	0	0	1	*	*	*	*
Tangerine, 2 med.	70	1	19	0	2	2	30	85	2	*
Watermelon, 2 cups cubed	80	1	19	0	1	10	8	25	*	2

*Less than 2 percent.

Source: Nutritional Labeling Data provided by the Food and Drug Administration and Food Processor II™.

weight due to the cravings and subsequent high-volume intake. It is hypothesized that it is a hormonal imbalance due to overproduction of insulin in the body.

It is now thought that insulin levels in our systems affect food cravings. In experiments, volunteers were hooked up to IVs through which insulin and glucose were added to their blood. In the placebo group, nothing changed. Throughout the procedure, their level of hunger did not increase. In the control group, however, the higher the amount of insulin that was added to the blood, the hungrier the person felt, and the more cravings they mentioned.

Now there are ways to keep this "disorder" under control. One way is to eat a nutritious diet while limiting the number of carbohydrates. To achieve balance, three meals per day or several smaller nutritious snacks per day are essential. Another regulator of insulin is an odd little trace mineral called chromium. This mineral is thought to be deficient in most of the population because it is lost in food processing. Taking supplements of this mineral should be done only with guidance from a health care professional. Regular exercise also seems to be important in stopping hyperinsulinemia because it seems to increase the number of insulin receptors in muscle cells, getting insulin out of the bloodstream. Without exercise, insulin remains in the bloodstream and can cause excessive hunger and other unpleasant symptoms.

To avoid food cravings, eat three sensible meals per day, get enough vitamins and minerals, control intake of high-carbohydrate foods, and exercise regularly. For the other basic components of a nutritious diet, refer to Chapters 5 and 6.

DIABETES AS A NATIONAL HEALTH PROBLEM

Diabetes has become a major American health problem. It has been documented as such not only in scientific publications, but lay magazines as well, in an attempt to get the attention of all Americans, so that we may begin as a nation to address this serious national health threat (Adler & Kalb, 2000).

Documenting the Problem

Dietary intake that includes too many calories from carbohydrates and fats contributes to the development diabetes. Abdominal obesity is associated with an increased risk of Type II diabetes when adjusting for body mass index, age, smoking, and alcohol consumption (Okosun, 2000).

Researchers have found that the common denominator in patients who develop adolescent-onset Type II diabetes is extreme obesity with body mass index (BMI) of 35–38 kg/m(2), accompanied by family obesity, a diet rich in fat, and a sedentary lifestyle. The current epidemic of Type II diabetes among adolescents demonstrates that failure to prevent obesity at primary and secondary opportunities for intervention leads to the development of associated diseases with significant morbidity and potential mortality (Pinhas-Hamiel & Zeitler, 2000).

Among college students who have Type I diabetes, most report that their disease is more difficult to handle at school than at home. Commonly reported barriers to diabetes control include diet, irregular schedules, lack of parental involvement, peer pressure, drugs and alcohol, fear of hypoglycemia, and finances. Factors identified as improving diabetes control are an increased sense of responsibility, increased frequency of blood glucose testing, exercise, contact with health care providers, fear of hyperglycemia, and knowledge of the results of the Diabetes Control and Complications Trial. Many students reported testing their blood more frequently and taking more injections than in high school; most were on intensive insulin regimens (Ramchandani et al., 2000).

One study found that men and women hold differing beliefs about ability to control their diabetes and degree of social support for diet, with males expressing stronger perceptions of control and social support for diet. The impact of gender differences on ability to integrate diabetes self-care and on effectiveness of diabetes programs has not been determined but should be considered in future research (Brown et al., 2000).

Combating the Problem

Whether metabolic control in Type II diabetes is best achieved with the traditional high-carbohydrate, low-fat diet or a low-carbohydrate, high-fat diet is still controversial. One study investigated the effect of using olive oil as the main edible fat in home meal preparation and found that such a diet is a good alternative diet to the traditional low-fat diet for patients with Type II diabetes (Rodriguez-Villar et al., 2000).

A reduction in the risk of diabetes among African American and Hispanic women could be possible by instituting public health measures for reducing waist size to the levels seen in white women. Intervention programs designed for reducing overall obesity and, consequently, waist size through lifestyle modification, including exercise and diet, may have considerable public health significance in reducing the incidence of Type II diabetes in these populations (Okosun, 2000).

Clinic- and community-based diabetes intervention programs have been found effective in improving dietary, physical activity, and self-care behaviors of older African American women with Type II diabetes. When designing programs it is important to construct them to be culturally relevant in order to be acceptable and effective (Keyserling et al., 2000).

SUMMARY

Carbohydrates are the most abundant and least expensive of all the food groups. Carbohydrates are found in sugar, fruits, vegetables, and grains, including bread and pasta, to name but a few sources. People often create problems for themselves by eating too many carbohydrates. Carbohydrate addiction and diabetes are examples of the problems that may develop in relation to excessive carbohydrate intake. There are numerous research reports to validate the role of foods in illness and solutions to help counteract the effects of diabetes.

REFERENCES

Adler, J., & Kalb, C. (2000, September 4). An American epidemic—Diabetes. *Newsweek, 136*(10), 40–47.

Brown, S. A., Harrist, R. B., Villagomez, E. T., Segura, M., Barton, S. A., & Hanis, C. L. (2000). Gender and treatment differences in knowledge, health beliefs, and metabolic control in Mexican Americans with type II diabetes. *Diabetes Education, 26*(3), 425–438.

Keyserling, T. C., Ammerman, A. S., Samuel-Hodge, C. D., Ingram, A. F., Skelly, A. H., Elasy, T. A., Johnston, L. F., Cole, A. S., & Henriquez-Roldan, C. F. (2000). A diabetes management program for African American women with type II diabetes. *Diabetes Education, 26*(5), 796–805.

Pinhas-Hamiel, O., & Zeitler, P. (2000) "Who is the wise man?—The one who foresees consequences": Childhood obesity, new associated comorbidity, and prevention. *Prevention Medicine, 31*(6), 702–705

Okosun, I. S. (2000). Ethnic differences in the risk of type II diabetes attributable to differences in abdominal adiposity in American women. *Journal of Cardiovascular Risk, 7*(6), 425–430.

Ramchandani, N., Cantey-Kiser, J. M., Alter, C. A., Brink, S. J., Yeager, S. D., Tamborlane, W. V., & Chipkin, S. R. (2000). Self-reported factors that affect glycemic control in college students with type I diabetes. *Diabetes Education, 26,* 656–666.

Rodriguez-Villar, C., Manzanares, J. M., Casals, E., Perez-Heras, A., Zambon, D., Gomis, R., & Ros, E. (2000). High-monounsaturated fat, olive oil–rich diet has effects similar to a high-carbohydrate diet on fasting and postprandial state and metabolic profiles of patients with type II diabetes. *Metabolism, 49*(12), 1511–1517.

Vitamins and Minerals

Do you or your clients need vitamin and mineral supplements? The vitamin controversy has been flaming for years. Ever since we learned about the relationship between nutrients and disease, we have wondered if supplements can take the place of or augment food. The fact is that most Americans do not eat the types of foods necessary to ensure optimal amounts of essential vitamins and minerals. Reliance on highly processed products, strict dieting, or high-stress lifestyles can inadvertently lead to nutritional deficiencies.

VITAMINS

Vitamins were first recognized as vital to the maintenance of good health in 1906. By 1915, a fat-soluble food factor was extracted from butter, egg yolks, and fish liver, while a water-soluble food factor was extracted from rice bran. In 1920, in order to distinguish the two, the fat-soluble factor was called *vitamin A* and the water-soluble factor, *vitamin B*. In 1956 more factors were isolated and identified from the original vitamin B "antiberiberi group," so numbers were added to the letter to further differentiate them. As other types of vitamins were discovered, they were assigned letters such as vitamins C, D, E, and so on.

What Are Vitamins?

Vitamins are organic (carbon-containing) molecules that are necessary for growth and maintenance of life. Vitamins must be obtained from the foods we eat or taken as supplements. An exception to this is vitamin D, which can be obtained from eating but more frequently is activated in the skin during exposure to sunlight. Although they are often connected with energy, vitamins provide none themselves but rather speed up the chemical reactions that the body does use for energy.

Vitamins also facilitate the reactions leading to repair and other processes essential to life. The absence of a vitamin will prevent the completion of a reaction, resulting in tissue damage that manifests where the vitamin is most active. For instance, a deficiency of B_2 shows up as cracking at the corners of the mouth and lips, a lack of vitamin A causes night blindness, and a vitamin D deficiency manifests itself as rickets. Prolonged absence of a vitamin may result in a serious illness. Most often, a malfunction involves a number of nutrients instead of one isolated factor since vitamins work together to perform tasks. Therefore, the use of complexes or multivitamins may be more beneficial since it can be difficult to isolate the weak links.

FAT-SOLUBLE VITAMINS

Vitamins that concentrate in fatty tissues and cell membranes, such as A, D, E, and K, need fat for proper assimilation. On the other hand, because they can be stored in these areas and in the liver, toxic level buildup is possible.

WATER-SOLUBLE VITAMINS

Vitamins such as B and C are carried by the blood throughout the body and are absorbed by the cells where they are needed. They must be replenished every day from food and, if needed, from supplements because they cannot be stored in the body. Any excess is excreted in the urine, although large amounts of an isolated vitamin may create an imbalance if used indiscriminately without adequate knowledge or guidance.

How Much Do We Need?

Supplement labels list the percentage of the U.S. RDA/DRI for the particular vitamin within the formula. Because the RDA/DRI applies to presumably healthy people, no special considerations are given for people with metabolic disorders, severe infections, chronic illnesses, certain environmental conditions, or varying lifestyles. Many people can exist on the U.S. RDAs/DRIs, while others find the vitamin recommendations too low. Higher potencies are warranted for some conditions; substances should be used with discretion and preferably some guidance. Table 8–1 (on pages 98–100) lists some of the more common vitamins. Some are listed without RDAs/DRIs because of insufficient knowledge about the exact levels needed or because their status as a true vitamin is questioned by the

National Academy of Sciences. Dosages for vitamins B, C, and K are expressed in terms of weight, milligrams (mg) or micrograms (mcg), while vitamins A, D, and E are stated in units of activity, international units (i.u.). International units are used with vitamin E instead of milligrams or micrograms to standardize the many forms of E available.

Vitamins As Antioxidants

Among the fastest selling of all vitamins are the antioxidants: vitamins C, E, and beta-carotene. A decade of laboratory research has shown that it is oxidation that makes cholesterol so harmful to coronary arteries. Although only a few human studies have been published, the results indicate that low levels of these vitamins correlate with a higher death rate from heart disease. Findings point to the fact that certain doses of antioxidant supplements can reduce the risk of myocardial infarction by one-half among men with histories of cardiovascular disease. The only side effect found so far is that excessive quantities of vitamin C may cause diarrhea or stomach distress, but since it is water-soluble and expelled in the urine, overdose is not a danger, with the rare exception of the development of renal stones. Vitamin E and beta-carotene can accumulate in our fat stores, but the side effects of this are no more serious than a stomachache or yellowing of the skin, which is reversible with time.

Simply stated, antioxidants work as follows:

1. A normal oxygen atom has four pairs of electrons. Through aging and general wear and tear on our systems, metabolism can take one of the electrons away from the atom. This changes the composition of the oxygen molecule and it becomes a "free radical." This new free radical then attempts to replace its lost electron by attacking other molecules.

2. When the free radical attacks and robs an electron from another molecule in the cell wall, a new free radical is created. A chain reaction begins when this newly created free radical seeks to take an electron from yet another molecule.

3. The chain of electron theft begins to erode the cell membrane and leads to disintegration of the cell. When this occurs, the cell surface is exposed to cancerous changes or a host of other ills.

4. The antioxidants have particular molecular structures. Because of their structure, they can go to the tissue and give up their electrons without becoming harmful and invading other cells. Thus, the chain reaction that culminates in cell-wall disintegration is aborted.

In essence, the antioxidant vitamins C, E, and beta-carotene may control the harmful free radical molecules and thereby prevent many common diseases.

TABLE 8–1 Vitamin Information

VITAMIN AND U.S. RDA/DRI LEVEL	FUNCTION	FOOD SOURCES	DEFICIENCY SYMPTOMS
B₁ (Thiamine) 1.5 mg	Needed for carbohydrate digestion, growth in children, and maintenance of organ muscle tone. Vital for a healthy nervous system and mental health and linked to improved learning capacity.	Wheat germ, bran, whole grains, blackstrap molasses, nutritional yeast	Easy fatigue, irritability, loss of appetite, constipation, mental depression.
B₂ (Riboflavin) 1.8 mg	Necessary for cell respiration, food metabolism, maintenance of healthy eyes, skin, and mouth.	Liver, tongue, organ meats, egg yolks, milk, cheese, wheat germ	Cracked lips and corners of mouth, inflammation of mouth, swollen tongue, itching, burning, bloodshot eyes, dizziness, sensitivity to light.
B₃ (Niacin) 20 mg	Acts as a coenzyme in digestion, dilates blood vessels, improves circulation, reduces cholesterol in blood. Needed for healthy skin, proper functioning of nervous system, and production of sex hormones.	Lean meats, poultry, fish, peanuts, wheat germ, nutritional yeast	Muscle weakness, fatigue, insomnia, irritability, canker sores, gastrointestinal disturbances, and recurring headaches.
B₆ (Pyridoxine) 2.0 mg	Needed for production of antibodies and red blood cells, aids digestion, promotes normal functioning of nervous and musculoskeletal systems, reduces cholesterol level in the bloodstream.	Bananas, wheat germ, leafy greens, raw meats, milk	Low blood sugar, nervousness, hair loss, muscle cramps, water retention, and nausea in pregnancy.
Biotin 300 mcg	Metabolism of fats, production of fatty acids, food metabolism, and the utilization of other B vitamins.	Found in all animal and plant tissue and traces are present in most whole foods, liver, legumes, egg yolk, meats	Muscular pain, exhaustion, loss of appetite, and depression.
Choline (none stated)	Fat metabolism, cholesterol utilization, normal nerve transmission. Essential for health of liver, kidneys, and the production of thyroid hormones.	Wheat germ, lecithin, yeast, egg yolks, liver, whole grains	Fatty deposits in liver, bleeding ulcers, kidney problems, high blood pressure. Prolonged deficiency can result in cirrhosis of the liver and atherosclerosis.

VITAMIN AND U.S. RDA/DRI LEVEL	FUNCTION	FOOD SOURCES	DEFICIENCY SYMPTOMS
Inositol (none stated)	Metabolism of fats and reduction of blood cholesterol, formation of lecithin in the body. Vital for hair growth and brain cell nutrition.	Citrus fruits, whole grains, yeast, liver, milk	Constipation, eczema, eye problems, hair loss, high blood serum cholesterol.
Folic Acid 400 mcg	Formation of red blood cells, cell growth and reproduction, health of the liver, hair, and scalp.	Green leafy vegetables, liver, whole grains, oysters, nutritional yeast	Gastrointestinal disturbances, hair loss or graying, tongue inflammation, anemia, toxemia in pregnancy.
Pantothenic Acid 10 mg	Stimulation of adrenal glands, utilization of other vitamins, building of body cells, resistance to stress, formation of antibodies and maintenance of normal digestive functions.	Organ meats, egg yolks, nutritional yeast, whole grains, green vegetables, royal jelly	Digestive problems, hypoglycemia, allergies, upper respiratory infections, burning or tingling feet and skin disorders.
Paba (Para Aminobenzoic Acid) (none stated)	Occurs in combination with folic acid. Promotes red blood cell formation, healthy skin, can restore color to gray hair, creates a natural sunscreen, promotes healthy intestinal flora.	Liver, nutritional yeast, wheat germ, milk, eggs, organ meats, blackstrap molasses	Constipation and digestive problems, extreme fatigue, headache, loss of hair color and skin pigmentation.\n\nSulfa drugs destroy paba.
B₁₂ (Cyanocobalamin) 6 mcg	Construction and regeneration of red blood cells, anti-anemia factor, food metabolism, healthy nervous system.	Liver, meat, fish, milk, eggs, yogurt, miso, pollen, wheat germ	Extreme fatigue, anemia, brain damage, nervous system disorders. Symptoms may take 5 or 6 years to appear.
B₁₅ (Pangamic Acid) (none stated)	Promotes cell respiration, antioxidant, regulates fat and sugar metabolism, and is essential in protein metabolism, particularly in heart muscle. Stimulates immune responses.	Nutritional yeast, brown rice, whole grains, pumpkin, and sesame seeds	Glandular and nervous disorders, heart disease.
C 60 mg	Helps prevent infections, strengthens connective tissues, healthy teeth, gums, bones. Promotes healing, maintains integrity of capillaries, collagen production, antioxidant.	Citrus fruits, tomatoes, green peppers, strawberries, kale, broccoli, parsley, most fresh fruits and vegetables	Bleeding gums, tooth decay, weak capillaries, bruising easily, nosebleeds, lowered resistance to infection, slow healing.

(continued)

99

TABLE 8–1 Vitamin Information (continued)

VITAMIN AND U.S. RDA/DRI LEVEL	FUNCTION	FOOD SOURCES	DEFICIENCY SYMPTOMS
A 5,000 i.u.	Ensures normal structure and function of cell membranes, acts to fight infection and build disease resistance necessary for healthy skin, bone, and teeth formation. Essential for the formation of visual purple, which is necessary for night vision.	Eggs, liver, dairy products, carrots, green leafy vegetables, colored fruits and vegetables	Night blindness; acne; dry, scaly skin; tooth decay; increased susceptibility to infection.
D 400 i.u.	Proper formation of bones and teeth, thyroid function, normal blood clotting, assimilation of calcium and phosphorus.	Milk, eggs, sardines, salmon, tuna	Tooth decay, pyorrhea, muscular weakness, porous bones, bone disorders–rickets in children, osteomalacia in adults.
E 30 i.u.	Improves circulation, promotes longevity, antioxidant, prevents blood clots, strengthens capillary walls, aids healing, promotes healthy skin and reproductive organs.	Wheat germ, nuts, seeds, cold pressed vegetable oils, organ meats	Sterility, miscarriage, heart disease, enlarged prostate, strokes, liver damage.
F (Unsaturated Fatty Acids) (none stated)	Promotes growth, healthy hair and skin, normal glandular activity, destroys cholesterol, helps prevent atherosclerosis, maintains body lubrication.	Butter, wheat germ, vegetable oils, sunflower seeds	Acne, dandruff, eczema, varicose veins, diarrhea, weak nails, underweight.
K (Phylioquinone) (none stated)	Promotes proper blood clotting, healthy liver function, longevity.	Eggs, soy oil, kelp, yogurt, leafy green vegetables, cauliflower	Nosebleeds, miscarriages, hemorrhaging due to improper clotting, intestinal malabsorption, diarrhea.
P (Bioflavonoids, Rutin, Hesperidin) (none stated)	Prevents infection, promotes healthy capillary walls and connective tissue, prevents bruising, aids in absorption of vitamin C.	White rind in fruits, cherries, black currants, buckwheat	Bruising easily, bleeding easily, low resistance to infection, varicose veins.

MINERALS

Minerals, one of the most understated classes of nutrients, are finally getting the status they deserve. We are only now beginning to recognize the importance of minerals. For one thing, without minerals, vitamins cannot be assimilated or utilized by the body.

What Are They?

Minerals are used by our bodies to form bones, teeth, soft tissue, muscles, blood, and nerve cells. Besides functioning as structural components, minerals are also catalysts for many reactions within the body, such as transmission of nerve impulses, digestion, and muscle response. In addition, they assist in producing hormones, maintaining the acid/alkaline balance in our bodies, and manufacturing antibodies.

What Foods Have Them?

Highly assimilated organic minerals are found in fruits and vegetables from the soil or sea or from fish or animals whose mineral content originates from eating land or sea plants. A varied diet containing whole grains, beans, nuts and seeds, leafy greens, fruits, and, if desired, dairy products, meat, poultry, fish, and eggs has the potential to provide all the minerals we need. Refined sugars and carbohydrates should be minimized since they retain very few minerals originally present in the food.

How Much Do We Need?

Calcium, chlorine, phosphorus, potassium, magnesium, sodium, and sulfur are called macrominerals because relatively large amounts are needed in the body. Zinc, iron, manganese, copper, chromium, selenium, iodine, and molybdenum are referred to as trace minerals because only minute amounts are required. Although most minerals have a general U.S. RDA/DRI established value, trace minerals have a significantly narrow margin of safety. It is easy to take too much, develop toxicity, and create a deficiency in another trace mineral. Unless proper levels of minerals are maintained and monitored, the delicate mineral balance of our bodies can be upset.

Chelated Minerals

Our bodies must convert inorganic minerals from the earth, such as dolomite, oyster shell, egg shell, and bone meal, into an organic form that we can assimilate. A chelated mineral is bound to another substance such as gluconic acid from corn (glyconates), lactic acid from milk or corn (lactates), fumaric acid from plants (fumerates), sulfuric acid (sulfates), ascorbic acid (ascorbates, citric acid, citrates), amino acids from soy or milk protein (amino acid chelates), or orotic acid (oratates).

Table 8–2 (on pages 104–105) details mineral information. Note that some minerals are listed without RDAs/DRIs because there is insufficient knowledge about the exact levels needed.

VITAMIN AND MINERAL SUPPLEMENTS

Ideally, we should be able to rely on natural foods to supply all the nutrients we need to maintain optimum health. However, where and how the food is grown; how it is processed, transported, and stored; and how old it is when we eat it all affect the nutrient value of food. In addition to the food factors themselves, age, heredity, environment, activity level, stress, and lifestyle determine how we assimilate nutrients and how much of each one we need.

Common Terms

When reading labels or counseling clients about vitamins and minerals, it is important to know the meaning of the terminology. The following words are commonly used.

HYPOALLERGENIC

Denotes that a supplement contains none or few of the foods or substances constituting the most common sensitivities experienced by people. In most cases, the supplement will also be free of artificial flavor, colors, and preservatives.

INTERNATIONAL UNITS (I.U.)

Dosages of vitamins A, D, and E are stated in units of activity rather than weight. International units are used with vitamin E instead of milligrams or micrograms to standardize the many forms of vitamin E available. Their use with vitamins A and D is due simply to historical usage.

SUSTAINED RELEASE OR TIMED-RELEASE SUPPLEMENTS

These are designed to provide nutrients over a 6- to 12-hour period when frequent doses are not taken. Effectiveness varies with the manufacturer and the digestive system of the person taking the supplement.

U.S. RECOMMENDED DIETARY ALLOWANCE (U.S. RDA/DRI)

Estimates established by the Federal Drug Administration (FDA) to ensure against deficiencies in healthy people.

VEGETARIAN SUPPLEMENTS

Supplements that are free of any animal products or derivatives. They are sold as tablets, powders, or liquids; capsules are usually avoided because of beef gelatin source.

Natural versus Synthetic

A truly natural supplement is one that is a concentrated food source. Vitamins A and D are natural if they are derived from fish liver oil, alfalfa, rose hips, brewer's yeast, wheat germ oil, lecithin, or desiccated liver. Natural vitamin E sources are soy oil, bone meal, chlorophyll, aloe vera, evening primrose oil, and spirulina. However, many supplements are derived from a synthetic source, a laboratory product whose molecular structure is similar to the supplement being copied. Synthetic supplements are used because of the advantages of synthetic over natural in terms of cost, availability of a natural commercial source, size limitations on the pill itself, and the number of pills required for a certain potency.

Vitamins from a natural source can be concentrated only to a certain degree. Most B and C supplements are at least partially synthetic to provide quantities that can be used to offset a deficiency. However, it is possible to concentrate high potencies of vitamins A, D, and E from the natural sources. Natural sources can be beneficial because they may contain synergistic elements, naturally occurring coenzymes, and other vitamins and minerals that facilitate assimilation in our bodies. Many companies add a natural base to their synthetic supplements in order to provide the best results. In contrast, some people prefer to use pure synthetic supplements to avoid natural substances to which they are allergic or sensitive.

Both natural-source and synthetic-source supplements work well. Vitamin E is the only vitamin that is definitely recognized to be more effective in the natural state. Personal preference and the potency required are the determining factors in choosing a natural or synthetic supplement. If you require only minimal amounts to supplement your diet, natural supplements may be suitable. If you need higher potencies to offset a deficiency or if you have food sensitivities, you may want a synthetic-based supplement.

TABLE 8-2 Mineral Information

MINERAL AND U.S. RDA LEVEL FOR ADULTS & CHILDREN OVER 4	FUNCTION	FOOD SOURCES	DEFICIENCY SYMPTOMS
Calcium 800 mg 1,200–1,500 for older women	Builds bones and teeth and maintains bone density and strength. Helps prevent osteoporosis. Plays a role in regulating heartbeat, blood clotting, and muscle contraction.	Milk and milk products, sardines and salmon eaten with bones, dark green leafy vegetables, shellfish, sea vegetables, tempeh, rutabagas	Rickets in children, osteoporosis in adults.
Chloride 700–5,100 mg No RDA established	Maintains normal fluid shifts, balances pH of blood, forms hydrochloric acid in stomach.	Table salt, fish, pickled and smoked foods	Upset balance of acids and bases in body fluids (rare).
Chromium 0.03–0.20 mg No RDA established	Important for glucose metabolism; may be a cofactor for insulin.	Meat, cheese, whole grains, dried peas and beans, peanuts, brewer's yeast	Diabeteslike symptoms.
Copper 2 mg No RDA established	Formation of red blood cells, cofactor in absorbing iron into blood, helps in production of several enzymes involved in respiration, interacts with zinc.	Organ meats, shellfish, nuts, dried legumes, raisins, mushrooms	Rarely seen in adults. Infants: hypochronic anemia with abnormal development of bone, nervous tissue, lungs and pigmentation of hair.
Fluorine 1–4.0 mg No RDA established	Contributes to solid bone and tooth formation; may help prevent osteoporosis in adults.	Naturally or artificially fluoridated water, some kinds of black tea	Higher frequency of tooth decay.
Iodine 0.15 mg	Necessary for normal function of thyroid gland, essential for normal cell function, prevents goiter.	Sea vegetables, iodized salt, seafood, plants grown in iodine-rich soil	Thyroid enlargement (goiter). Newborns: cretinism.
Iron 10 mg (male) 18 mg (female)	Essential to formation of hemoglobin –the oxygen-carrying factor in the blood– and myoglobin–which stores oxygen in muscles.	Liver, meat products, egg yolk, shellfish, green leafy vegetables, legumes, whole grains, dried fruits	Iron deficiency anemia, pallor of skin, weakness and fatigue, headache, shortness of breath.

MINERAL AND U.S. RDA LEVEL FOR ADULTS & CHILDREN OVER 4	FUNCTION	FOOD SOURCES	DEFICIENCY SYMPTOMS
Magnesium 200–300 mg	Aids in bone growth, nerve conduction, muscle relaxation, regulation of normal heart rhythm, bowel function.	Nuts, legumes, whole grains, bananas, apricots, dark leafy greens	Muscular tremors, twitching, and weakness. Deficiency is sometimes seen in people with severe disease, prolonged diarrhea, or alcoholism.
Manganese 1.5–5.0 mg	Required for normal bone growth and development, part of some enzymes.	Nuts, whole grains, legumes, nonleafy vegetables, fruits, tea	Not well defined in humans.
Molybdenum 0.06–5.0 mg No RDA established	Enzyme constituent.	Whole grains, legumes, organ meats, dark green vegetables	Unknown in humans.
Phosphorus 800 mg	With calcium helps build strong bones and teeth. Needed by certain enzymes that help change food into energy.	Meat, poultry, fish, eggs, legumes, milk and milk products, whole grains	Weakness, bone pain, neurological problems (rare).
Potassium 775–5,624 mg	With sodium helps regulate body-fluid balance, transmission of nerve impulses, active in muscle contraction, promotes regular heartbeat.	Most fruits, starchy root vegetables, dark leafy green vegetables, peanut butter	Muscular weakness, irritability, irregular heartbeat.
Selenium 0.03–0.20 mg No RDA established	Cellular antioxidant, essential constituent of red blood cells and enzymes; decreases the toxicity of heavy metals, may inhibit cancer initiation.	Fish, shellfish, chicken, egg yolks, garlic, whole grains	Heart muscle damage, hemolytic anemia.
Sodium 450–3,300 mg No RDA established	Helps maintain water balance inside and outside cells, plays a role in maintaining blood pressure.	Salt, processed foods, ham, pickles, smoked foods	Muscle weakness, cramps, confusion, apathy, anorexia, low blood pressure.
Zinc 10–15 mg	Essential for more than 100 enzymes involved in growth, sexual maturation, wound healing, ability to taste, protein synthesis, immunity.	Meats, eggs, oysters, crabmeat, nuts, wheat germ	Loss of taste, delayed wound healing, growth retardation and delayed sexual maturation in children.

How Much Do We Need?

Most of the food labels on the shelves today are based on RDAs set in 1968. The FDA will not add new vitamin numbers to their recommendations until new reports are issued on how much protein, fat, and fiber we should eat.

Abundant information is available on the Internet. The U.S. Agriculture Department (USDA) has a clearinghouse of information for those interested in the many specific details of vitamins, minerals, and other components. Once you decide just how many nutrients you or your clients need, the USDA Internet site (http://www.nal.usda.gov/fnic/foodcomp) quickly shows descriptive data. For example, the site will tell you that a handful of almonds yields 7.5 milligrams of vitamin E, half a day's supply in a single snack. The American Dietetic Association (ADA) also provides information about food and nutrition and posts opinions and recommendations on the Positions Index of its Web site.

With a good foundation of a balanced diet, plenty of exercise, and adequate sleep, supplements can be an effective booster if more nutrients are actually needed. However, without test results and professional guidance, it is difficult to know what and how much to take. Pregnant and lactating women, heavy drinkers, women on oral contraceptives, and those who are unable to get an adequate diet due to a prolonged illness, digestive disorders, physical or emotional problems, or dieting can find it difficult to get all the nutrients they need from food. In these cases, supplements are beneficial.

Using the standards of the U.S. RDAs as general guidelines, many people start with a low-potency multiple vitamin/mineral supplement to cover most of the available nutrients in a balanced ratio. Keep in mind that more is not always better. The toxicity symptoms of a nutrient are sometimes similar to the deficiency symptoms and isolated doses of one nutrient may cause an imbalance. Higher potencies are warranted for some conditions, but they should be used with discretion and preferably under guidance.

When and How to Take Supplements

Fat-soluble supplements should be taken with foods to enhance absorption and to prevent nausea. If taken once a day, take them with the largest meal, preferably earlier in the day to avoid the stimulation that sometimes interferes with sleep. Water-soluble vitamins can be taken between meals. Calcium is better absorbed when taken with meals. However, foods high in iron compete for absorption in the small intestine.

Storage

Without preservation, supplements will keep 2 to 3 years if the bottle is unopened. Once opened, they will keep up to 1 year. Store in a cool, dry place away from sunlight. Do not store in the refrigerator because moisture builds up inside the bottle with constant opening and closing. Some companies add a silica gel packet to absorb excess moisture. A few grains of rice added to the bottle will give similar results.

Forms of Supplements

Supplements are available in many forms to facilitate the particular absorption requirements of the various nutrients and to provide alternatives for individual needs and desires.

TABLETS

These are the most familiar form and are easily stored. They usually require the addition of fillers and binders to form the tablet from loose material. High-pressure compression and coatings protect the tablets from moisture and facilitate swallowing. Some tablets are so compact that some people may have difficulty with absorption and utilization.

CHEWABLE TABLETS

These are most often sweetened with sugar, honey, molasses, fructose, or fruit concentrates. They are easy to take and are generally well-absorbed. The sugar content can be quite high, so if sugar is to be avoided, use powders, liquids, or capsules.

POWDERS AND LIQUIDS

These forms are very well assimilated and are usually quite potent. They can be mixed into liquids, foods, or taken by the spoonful. Unpalatable combinations generally are sweetened or flavored.

CAPSULES

These are usually well assimilated, easy to swallow, and tasteless. Capsules are not suitable for strict vegetarians because they are made from animal gelatin. Vegetarians and those who are allergic to beef can open the capsule, swallow the contents, and discard the capsule.

Potential Problems from Supplements

Some supplements can cause problems. It behooves health care professionals to be aware that the supplements industry is new and is still under scientific scrutiny.

For example, the supplements glucosamine and chondroitin sulfate have shown efficacy in relieving pain associated with osteoarthritis. However, evidence is limited concerning the chondroprotective ability of these agents. More controlled studies and basic research is necessary to evaluate these claims especially because these compounds are not under regulatory control (Callaghan, Buckwalter, & Schenck, 2000).

Not all supplements are vitamins, but many people take them as if they were. One of the popular supplements is blue-green algae (BGA). The presence of BGA toxins in surface waters used for drinking water sources and recreation is receiving increasing attention around the world as a public health concern. However, potential risks from exposure to these toxins in contaminated health food products that contain BGA have been largely ignored. BGA products are commonly consumed in the United States, Canada, and Europe for their putative beneficial effects, including increased energy and elevated mood. Many of these products contain *Aphanizomenon flos-aquae,* a BGA that is harvested from Upper Klamath Lake in southern Oregon, where the growth of a toxic BGA, *Microcystis aeruginosa,* is a regular occurrence. *M. aeruginosa* produces compounds called microcystins, which are potent hepatotoxins and probable tumor promoters. Because *M. aeruginosa* coexists with *A. flos-aquae,* it can be collected inadvertently during the harvesting process, resulting in microcystin contamination of BGA products. In fall 1996, the Oregon Health Division learned that Upper Klamath Lake was experiencing an extensive *M. aeruginosa* bloom, and an advisory was issued recommending against water contact. The advisory prompted calls from consumers of BGA products, who expressed concern about possible contamination of these products with microcystins. In response, the Oregon Health Division and the Oregon Department of Agriculture established a regulatory limit of 1 mg/g for microcystins in BGA-containing products and tested BGA products for the presence of microcystins. Microcystins were detected in 85 of 87 samples tested, with 63 samples (72 percent) containing concentrations over 1 mg/g (Gilroy, Kauffman, Hall, Huang, & Chu, 2000).

One research study was done to gain a better understanding of health food store personnel's recommendations to customers, in this study case, breast cancer patient care. A researcher posing as the daughter of a breast cancer patient surveyed personnel at 40 health food stores on their product recommendations for cancer care, including products and services, proposed mechanism of action, and costs. Store personnel readily provided information and product recommendations, with shark cartilage being the most frequent. Suggested mechanisms of action drew on traditional healing, scientific, and pseudoscientific rationales. Costs for recommended dosages varied widely across stores and brands. Retailers supplying supplements can play an important role in the network of "authorities" for patients with breast and other cancers, as they readily provide advice and recommend products. The reasons why patients seek health food store remedies are useful in developing approaches to patient education (Gotay & Dumitriu, 2000).

Health care providers are in a key position to assist cancer patients in making informed choices when considering health food store products.

SUMMARY

We have learned a great deal about vitamins and minerals since they were first recognized in the early 1900s. We need both water-soluble and fat-soluble vitamins, and should get the majority of them from the food we eat rather than relying solely on supplements. Supplements are valuable, but should be used with caution by recognizing that we are still acquiring the scientific data necessary to know which ones provide benefits and in what quantities and forms. Understanding their importance as we do now, we should ascertain our own needs and our clients' needs for adequate vitamin intake. Knowing that the length of time of body storage varies from one vitamin to another, we should maintain a diet filled with nutritious foods.

REFERENCES

Callaghan, J. J., Buckwalter, J. A., & Schenck, R. C. Jr. (2000, December). Argument against use of food additives for osteoarthritis of the hip. *Clinical Orthopedics* (381), 88–90.

Gilroy, D. J., Kauffman, K. W., Hall, R. A., Huang, X., & Chu, F. S. (2000). Assessing potential health risks from microcystin toxins in blue-green algae dietary supplements. *Environmental Health Perspectives, 108*(5), 435–439.

Gotay, C. C., & Dumitriu, D. (2000). Health food store recommendations for breast cancer patients. *Archives of Family Medicine, 9*(8), 692–699.

Emotions and Food

OVERVIEW

We all know the power of emotions. Sometimes they consume us, and sometimes we have them under control, but they are always with us. How we deal with the relationship between food and emotions is a significant part of who we are and how we respond.

CASE STUDY: Sarah

Sarah sat with her knee skinned and her head throbbing. She had fallen off her bicycle again. Soon Mother came out to hold and cuddle her and to put a bandage on that little cut—and to give her an ice cream cone to cheer her up.

Twenty years later, Sarah's pride is skinned and her head is throbbing. In the last year, she has gone through a divorce, been in a car accident, and lost her job. On top of all of this, she has gained nearly 40 pounds.

THE INTERTWINING RELATIONSHIP

Food and emotions are intertwined. From the time we are children, we are taken out to dinner for rewards, served ice cream when we hurt, and given pizza to celebrate. Virtually all of our happy holidays are filled with food. We have, in essence, become a society where food is all-important. Who has ever heard of a social gathering without the hors d'oeuvres or Thanksgiving with no turkey and dressing? We probably cannot imagine having a really happy time without food being included in some way. Even when we go to the movies, we are tempted by popcorn and candy.

As we consider the relationship between emotions and food, let us look at Sarah. When Sarah was a child and was hurt and given ice cream, she felt much better. Why? Because ice cream was a special treat, something that her mother gave her to cheer her up and take the sting out of the hurt. Falling off her bike did not mean that she was a failure. To prove it, she was given a reward.

Twenty years later, Sarah is still a good person. To prove that to herself, despite the failed marriage, she rewards herself with lots of delicious foods. Thus, a vicious cycle begins. The causative emotions in this instance are sadness and hurt. This probably results in reduced self-esteem. Going through a divorce is hard, but making herself a big plate of steaming hot, high-calorie food not only reassures Sarah, it is also delicious and warm. Even though she did not succeed in her marriage or in her job, food still tastes good and makes her feel better.

CASE STUDY: Larry

Larry jumped up and laughed. He had just received one of the top Scholastic Aptitude Test (SAT) scores in the nation. His parents, who were proud and happy for him, took him out to dinner where he ate his fill with a smile on his lips. Later when he got accepted into medical school, his parents threw him a dinner party one night, and he and his friends celebrated with pizza the next.

Ten years later, Larry is getting sued for malpractice. His wife and children stand by him supportively, but nothing seems to help. He knows that he has done nothing wrong; he has done his best. Despite how he tries, he cannot bring himself to have even a bite of the wonderful dinner his wife has prepared for him. He can tell she is worried about his weight loss during the past month, but somehow he feels much too sad to even touch his food. What if the malpractice suit goes to court?

Emotional Links

We know that there is a link between emotions and food. We need food to live, not just physically it seems, but emotionally. If we are at a comfortable weight, there is nothing wrong with rewarding ourselves with an occasional treat. Some of us, though, need food to feel happy or reassured.

In Larry's case food has served as a reward. When he was happy he ate, when he won something he ate, when things where going well he was able to eat. Yet, when he most needs the vitamins and minerals, he cannot even bring himself to touch food. For many, food is a psychologist. The problem, however, is that this food "psychologist" can cause trouble when we go to it for reassurance, as Sarah and Larry found. In Sarah's case, it caused her to put on weight. This made her feel more depressed, which led her to eat again. In Larry's case, he ate when he was succeeding or doing well, but when he really needed food, he rejected it.

Indulging ourselves occasionally if we are happy and maintain a healthy weight is fine, but food can become a problem when we link it too heavily with emotions.

ANGER

Anger is an emotion that we have all experienced. Hate and anger are strongly related and often cause the same problems, and one of those problems is with food.

CASE STUDY: Tina

While I was preparing to attend a dinner party, I got a frantic call from my friend, Tina. She was out of breath and upset because her son had taken their car without telling her, and she had no way to get to the party. We agreed that my husband and I would pick her up.

Tina looked good; she was wearing black to downplay the weight she had gained in the last year. As Tina talked, I could tell she was furious. Her son had been staying out late and his grades were falling. When we sat down for dinner, Tina attacked her food.

After dinner, we drove Tina home. Her son had arrived home by then. I walked her to the door and she seemed much calmer. When she saw her son, she politely said that there was something they needed to discuss. Then they both sat down at the table, and I left. Later she told me that she had behaved calmly and rationally and that she and the boy had come up with a system for sharing the car.

(Continued on next page)

The point of this story is to see the connection between anger and food. Tina ripped her chicken entrée to shreds, devoured two baked potatoes, three helpings of green beans, and two pieces of cheesecake. She seemingly took her anger out on the food by eating it. Later, with a full stomach, she used her calmness with her son. She had previously learned that her anger with him did not get her anywhere except back to the refrigerator.

Observation

Anger is a very primitive emotion, yet we still need it. Anger should motivate us to take action. It should not cause us to pick up the phone and call for a pizza. For Tina, it should have let her know that she needed help with her son. She should have used her anger to ground him or to find a really good place to hide the car keys. Anger should be used to benefit us, not to cause a weight problem.

LOVE

Now that we have talked about negative emotions, let us consider a positive one, love. Love and food are quite a combination. Most of the time when people first fall in love the desire to eat is not very strong. Why? Because deep down our bodies know they would rather reproduce than have a piece of cheesecake. As time goes on, however, love turns more to companionship, and we enjoy sharing our meals with our partners. When we eat together, we need to help each other by picking out healthy foods. Then we can go home, cuddle up, and have some fun working off the calories together.

Love is an emotion we often feel for others but not enough for ourselves, especially concerning what we eat. If we really cared about ourselves, we would want to stay healthy by exercising and eating low-fat foods. The most important part of the emotion love is learning to feel it about ourselves.

HAPPINESS

Happiness is a positive emotion, but we do not gain or lose weight because we are happy or sad. We create weight problems when we use food to satisfy our emotions, to reward ourselves, to relieve stress, or to vent. When we allow our untethered emotions to rule us, some of us starve ourselves, while others become obese.

Let us refer back to Larry. Larry is basically a happy person, someone who loves a good meal. Yet with any sadness, he loses his will to eat. Larry is the type of person who does not care if food still tastes good, because his life is in torment. Larry still needs to eat, but food and emotion have become so linked in him that when he is unhappy, he loses his desire to eat.

In good times or in bad, we need to treat ourselves well. Take a long bath, see a good movie, and indulge in an occasional banana split. But just make sure the banana split includes a banana, and some low-fat frozen yogurt, and is topped with only a small portion of chocolate sauce. After the treat, take a walk and resolve the issue. By working with our emotions, we can benefit ourselves, not the local pizza parlor.

THE IMPORTANCE OF HOW WE EAT

How we eat is as important as what we eat. Many of us rush through our meals, gulping our food while paying little or no attention to what we are eating. We may be distracted by television, conversation, reading, or even daydreaming during our meals. The point is that we are not paying attention to our food. More often than not, when we eat like this, we gain weight, especially around midlife.

Many religious orders, both Western and Eastern, teach the importance of mindful eating. Mindful eating requires us to pay attention to what, with whom, how, when, where, and why we are eating. The theory behind mindful eating is that when we pause to reflect on the source, the preparation, the texture, the color, the shape, the arrangement, and so forth of the food item before us, we will better appreciate its value. As we consider the value of the food, we consider other aspects of its assimilation; for example, of what benefit is this food to us? How will this food make us stronger, healthier, or better able to perform? There is no question that these reflective questions better bind us to the food we eat and put us in a position to seriously consider what we are doing to and with our bodies. Attention to these questions constitutes the beginning phase of mindful eating.

To facilitate this exercise, begin by eating alone. Turn off the television and seat yourself in a comfortable setting. Examine the foods before you and think about the holistic aspects of each food item while you eat it. Calm your emotions. Think about the chewing process. Feel the foods and consider their effect on your body. As you practice this technique, notice how as you increase your attention to the food, you both decrease your speed and calm yourself.

After you have done this exercise alone a few times, try it in a group setting. It's best to begin with your family. Perhaps you will want to involve them in the process. You will probably notice that your speed of eating has slowed compared to others. As you gain skill in mindful eating, you will find that you can even eat mindfully in a group. You will probably find, however, that you are a little slower and probably calmer than your friends. Just remember, the idea is to completely nourish your body, mind, and spirit. Doing this requires mindfulness.

SUMMARY

Food and emotions are interrelated, but they need not be directly correlated to the extent that they rule our lives. Each day and every event give us opportunities to respond with positive, negative, and/or neutral emotions and to develop emotional self-control. Emotional balance can be achieved with conscious effort. When we discipline our emotions and achieve emotional harmony, we are in a superior position to develop healthy eating behaviors. One of the keys to vibrant health is to develop eating habits based on sensible, conscious choices rather than on the dictates of unconscious emotional drives.

CHAPTER 10

Nutrition through the Life Span

Nutritional needs vary throughout the life span. This chapter focuses on the differences that occur during the developmental, adult life, and receding years.

YOUTH

Infants

Milk is the first food for infants. It is now generally accepted that the mother's breast milk is the food of choice for babies from birth to weaning. Weaning age varies from person to person and culture to culture. For most babies, it is between 6 months to 1 year of age.

Formula-fed babies follow the specific regimens prescribed by their practitioners. Following the switch from formula to milk, it is important that skim milk not be used for infants. Skim milk lacks linoleic acid (an essential fatty acid) and has inadequate calories.

Introduction of solid foods should not begin until at least after 4 to 6 months of age because salivary amylase for the digestion of starches is not present until then. Cereals are usually introduced first. If the sweeter fruits are introduced first, the baby will reject the cereal in preference of the sweeter taste. Egg whites should not be offered until the baby is over 12 months because infants frequently develop allergies to the protein in egg whites before this age.

Preschool and School-Age Children

Overall, for children ages 2 to 12, it is very important to instill good eating habits and avoid overindulgence in refined sugars and flours and high-fat, fried fast foods. Children need a lot of nourishing foods to provide them with all of the important nutrients for growth; though physical growth is a little slower in this age period than it is in infancy or during adolescent years, mental growth is relatively rapid (Hass, 2000). Creating healthy eating patterns begins with encouraging the consumption of good quality, wholesome foods, which is a lot easier when parents eat this type of diet. Children's tendencies are toward the sweets, treats, and salted snacks and away from vegetables, the important food group that probably offers the greatest nutritional challenge for parents. Try to be creative with veggies; most children prefer raw vegetables to cooked, so try more raw veggies. Basically, offer whatever vegetables the children like and maintain the fruits, grains, and protein foods.

Many children like to help and be part of their nutrition. Support this by reaching agreements and creatively inspiring their food choices and by teaching them to prepare food and feed themselves at an early age. Avoid soft drinks and excessive, poor quality "treat" foods. Instead, offer more nourishing snacks, such as fruits, cheese or yogurt, crackers, and nuts or popcorn (if the children are older than four). Avoid nutritional adversity—those battles and hassles around mealtime that lead to rewards of sweets such as ice cream, cake, or candy, or just dessert, to children for eating their vegetables. Bribery and rewards may emphasize the treats and lessen the value of the more healthful foods. Again, getting children involved in meal planning and preparation as they get older is often helpful. Having them assist in preparing their school lunch will give them more identity with it and pleasure in eating it. Good eating habits will generate good nutrition and thus a good mind and good actions.

As insurance to prevent nutrient deficiencies, many parents want their children to take supplements. Chewables are still a favorite, though as they grow, many kids can swallow pills and capsules. Powdered formulas can be added to foods (Hass, 2000).

PRESCHOOL CHILDREN

Children from 1 to 3 years of age slow their rate of growth from that of infancy. They have a decreased appetite and consequent decrease in food consumption. During this time, they manifest a desire for independence and often will favor nonnutritious foods. From 3 to 6 years their requirements do not change much, but this is the time they observe others for eating habits and styles. If the parents eat nutritious foods, the child will probably follow. On the other hand, if the parents are fast-food junkies, the preschool-age child will likely emulate this style.

Keep their diet low in refined foods, chemical foods, and sweet, salty, or fried foods. At this age children like to eat with their hands, especially finger snacks, so give them small pieces at meals when appropriate.

SCHOOL-AGE CHILDREN

From 6 to 12 years, children grow slowly and steadily. Continued protein intake is important for muscle development, and milk intake is important for bone development. At this age, vitamin A and C deficiencies are common because many children do not have an adequate intake of the recommended quantities of fresh fruits and vegetables.

Often likes and dislikes will limit the diets of school-age children. Food games lose their charm, and rebellion may begin. On the other hand, many children in this age group will become more cooperative and want to be helpful and accepted and thus may really attempt to eat well. A good breakfast is essential for children going off to school. Eating hot, whole-grain cereals provides a good source of morning energy (sugary cereals may be more stimulating, but the boost is short-lived and may be followed by a depressed period); some protein, such as eggs, will also provide sustaining energy. It is important to remember that there are always outside influences on children this age, such as other children or television, that can undermine the healthful eating habits you have tried to develop in your children. Setting a good example is the best influence parents have on the overall nutritional patterns of their young ones (Hass, 2000).

Many parents overestimate their children's nutritional needs and the amount of food they require. It is best to create simple meals and serve smaller portions more frequently throughout the day. Needs for calories and many of the basic nutrients will vary from ages 2 through 10. Obviously, with increased size and activity, older children will need more food, which they naturally will eat. The more we can support them in avoiding empty calories, the better chance they will have of optimum growth. During the middle years, the average youngster will gain between five and eight pounds and grow about one-half inch per year, provided they have the nutrients they need. Support a healthy amount of physical activity in place of laziness or too much TV, telephone, and/or videogames.

Adolescents

Between the ages of 12 and 20, the rate of growth is greater than at any other period of life except infancy. Girls may add over 3 inches, and boys 4 or more inches in height. Because of this growth spurt, the need for calories will increase at some time during this period. Boys may need 2,700 to 2,900 calories per day, and girls will require 2,100 to 2,200 calories per day.

During this period, it is important to maintain sufficient protein intake. Boys need protein for the development of muscle mass and long bone growth, which are controlled by testosterone. Girls need protein for the synthesis of increased fat tissues and long bone growth.

The need for the minerals calcium and phosphorus is 50 percent higher than it is during childhood because of the increased bone growth. Iron is particularly important in girls to replace what is lost during menstruation and in boys for muscle development. Of course, all other vitamins and minerals must be consumed at the recommended levels.

ADULTS

The macronutrient needs of both men and women vary with age and sex as well as with physiological events and life habits. The role of nutrients such as antioxidants in the slowing of metabolic aging or reduction of the consequences of the stress have been widely stated in the media, yet scientifically established benefits are less well known. For example, the major role played by the antioxidants in the fight against opacity of lens and macular degeneration is just now being explored (Choay, 2000). The next section explores the many ways that nutrition relates to health for both women and men.

Women

Recent research demonstrates that consuming soy is beneficial for all women, but how much and from what foods are still under determination. It is important for health practitioners to be aware of the potential benefits of soy as many of their women patients will be asking about alternatives for hormone replacement therapy, such as soy consumption (Lindsay & Claywell, 1999).

For women of childbearing age, folates have a well-known preventive action on the abnormal closing of the neural tube, and reduce the risks of hypotrophy and premature births. Folates help reduce hyperhomocysteinemia, which in turn reduces risk for cardiovascular disease. As the benefits expected are documented and needed daily doses higher than those supplied by a balanced diet, or too often assumed as such, mineral-vitamin supplementation of women appears to be warranted (Choay, 2000).

Most women live longer than men. The life expectancy of women currently exceeds that of men by almost seven years, yet women spend approximately twice as many years disabled prior to death as their male counterparts. The diseases that account for death and health care utilization in older women (heart disease, cancer, stroke, fracture, pneumonia, osteoarthritis, cataracts) are also major contributors to disability (La Croix, Newton, Leveille, & Wallace, 1997). The need to emphasize prevention of coronary heart disease in women is important because first events are often fatal in women. Factors that are unique in terms of their influence on risk for coronary heart disease in women include age, reproductive and hormonal status, high density lipoprotein cholesterol and triglyceride levels, and the presence of diabetes (King & Mosca, 2000). A consistent plan to address risk factor management in individual women is the key to long-term risk reduction.

In every year since 1984, cardiovascular disease has claimed the lives of more females than males. More than 450,000 women succumb to heart disease annually, and 50,000 die of coronary artery disease (Giardina, 2000). Despite the facts, most women believe they will die of breast cancer. The misperception that heart disease is a man's disease and that women are more likely to die of breast cancer is alarming. Although women develop heart disease about 10 years later than men, they are likely to fare worse after a heart attack. The poorer outcomes are due, in part, to the failure to identify heart attack symptoms. Approximately 35 percent of heart attacks in women are believed to go unnoticed or unreported. However, because of increased age, women are more likely to have comorbid diseases such as diabetes and hypertension. In women, not only is tightness or discomfort in the chest a warning sign, but in addition, nausea and dizziness are common indicators of myocardial ischemia. Other symptoms include breathlessness, perspiration, a sensation of fluttering in the heart, and fullness in the chest.

In comparison to men, women are less likely to undergo tertiary care interventions such as cardiac catheterization, angioplasty, thrombolytic therapy, and bypass surgery; to participate in cardiac rehabilitation; and to return to work full-time after myocardial infarction. In the past, most research about treatments for heart disease focused on men, and gender differences have been ignored. Recent studies are enrolling enough women to test if there are differences between men and women in outcomes.

One of the major areas of research relates to estrogen and hormone replacement therapy to reduce the relative risk of heart attack and stroke. The Women's Health Initiative is a major study sponsored by the National Institutes of Health (NIH) that addresses the issue of primary prevention of cardiac disease by hormone replacement therapy. The results will be available in 2004. The Heart Estrogen/Progestin Replacement Study (HERS), disappointingly, did not show a significant reduction of coronary events in women taking hormone replacement therapy, nor did the Estrogen Replacement and Atherosclerosis (ERA) trial of 309 post-menopausal women who underwent coronary angiography. New insight into the role of vitamins, phytoestrogens and other natural sources, and selective estrogen receptor modulators may provide other options for management. Until then, modification of risk factors and healthy lifestyle choices are recommended for reducing the risk of cardiac disease. In fact, the key to a healthy heart appears closely tied to lifestyle choices. Prevention of disease is the key and current recommendations are simple: stop smoking or do not start; treat and control blood pressure (> 140/90 mm Hg); manage elevated lipids by diet, exercise, and cholesterol-lowering medications (if necessary); treat diabetes; lose weight so that your body mass index (BMI) is < 25; walk for 20 to 30 minutes at least three times a week; and take an aspirin tablet daily (Giardina, 2000).

There is scientific evidence to support specific recommendations for older women that may prevent or delay these conditions for as long as possible (La Croix et al., 1997). Whenever possible, health care providers will want to implement and encourage the following:

1. Assess risk factors for falls and fractures and, where possible, modify the environment to minimize occurrences.

2. Recommend adequate intake of calcium, vitamin D, fruits, and vegetables.

3. Encourage a weight management program for most women.

4. Screening for B_{12} deficiency is recommended for most women.

5. Engage women in a shared decision-making process about the use of hormone replacement therapy for long-term prevention of heart disease and fractures.

6. Encourage regular screening for breast and colorectal cancer.

7. Recommend enjoyable physical activities, including walking, for 30 minutes daily.

These interventions have the potential to delay the onset and improve the course of many chronic conditions that prevail in later life.

Biological, environmental, and social factors predispose women to cardiovascular diseases, malignancy, osteoporosis, diabetes, obesity, and eating disorders. Their prevention requires that health services recognize women as a risk group and provide appropriate financial and professional resources. To develop and apply intervention programs for women, funding must be allocated for data collection, development and assessment of intervention programs, and involving women in decision processes (Kaluski & Levental, 1999).

The Women's Health Initiative (WHI), established by the NIH in 1991, is a long-term national health study that focuses on strategies for preventing heart disease, breast and colorectal cancer, and osteoporosis in postmenopausal women. These chronic diseases are the major causes of death, disability, and frailty in older women of all races and socioeconomic backgrounds. The WHI is a 15-year multi-million-dollar endeavor, and is one of the most definitive, far-reaching clinical trials of women's health ever undertaken in the United States. Also one of the largest U.S. prevention studies of its kind, the WHI involves over 161,000 women ages 50 to 79. The WHI Clinical Trial and Observational Study attempts to address many of the inequities in women's health research and provide practical information to women and their physicians about hormone replacement therapy, dietary patterns and calcium/vitamin D supplements, and their effects on the prevention of heart disease, cancer, and osteoporosis. Emerging information from the WHI and other studies of women's health begun in the 1990s should change the landscape of options for older women in the years to come (McGowan & Pottern, 2000).

CURRENT RESEARCH STUDIES ON WOMEN AND NUTRITION

Several current scientific studies validate the importance of good nutrition to women's health. Prospective data relating fruit and vegetable intake to cardiovascular disease (CVD) risk are sparse, particularly for women. Thus in a large, prospective cohort of women, researchers examined the hypothesis that higher fruit and vegetable intake reduces CVD risk (Liu et al., 2000). They assessed fruit and vegetable intake among 39,876 female health professionals with no previous history of CVD or cancer using a detailed food-frequency questionnaire, and subsequently followed the women for an average of 5 years for incidence of nonfatal myocardial infarction (MI), stroke, percutaneous transluminal coronary angioplasty, coronary artery bypass graft, or death due to CVD. Participants with a self-reported history of diabetes, hypertension, or high cholesterol at baseline were excluded from the study. During follow-up, they documented 418 incident cases of CVD, including 126 MIs. After adjustment for age, randomized treatment status, and smoking, the researchers observed a significant inverse association between fruit and vegetable intake and CVD risk. An inverse, though not statistically significant, trend remained after additional adjustment for other known CVD risk factors. Higher fruit and vegetable intake also was associated with a lower risk of MI. These data suggest that higher intake of fruit and vegetables may be protective against CVD and support current dietary guidelines to increase fruit and vegetable intake (Liu et al., 2000).

Not all studies support the role of fruit and vegetable consumption as a preventative measure. In 1998 research was done to determine the role of fruit and vegetable consumption and dietary intake of folic acid and related nutrients such as methionine, cysteine, and alcohol in the etiology of breast cancer (Thorand, Kohlmeier, Simonsen, Croghan, & Thamm, 1998). In this study, dietary intake data were collected for 43 postmenopausal women diagnosed with breast cancer between 1991 and 1992 in Berlin, Germany, and compared to 106 population-based controls. Odds ratios adjusted for major risk factors of breast cancer, but not for total energy intake, showed a nonsignificant inverse association between a high intake of vegetables and fruits and breast cancer. Once results were adjusted for total energy intake the associations became much weaker. Alcohol intake was inversely associated with breast cancer in a nonsignificant way, possibly due to the relatively low alcohol intake of the study population. The results of this study do not provide firm evidence that a high intake of fruits and vegetables, folic acid, methionine, or cysteine reduces the risk of getting breast cancer (Thorand et al., 1998).

Antioxidant vitamins may play a role in the prevention of stroke because they scavenge free radicals and prevent LDL oxidation. Epidemiologic studies into this relation have produced conflicting results (Yochum, Folsom, & Kushi, 2000). One study of 34,492 postmenopausal women examined the association between antioxidant vitamin intake and death from stroke. During follow-up, 215 deaths from stroke were documented. Total vitamin A, carotenoid, and vitamin E intakes were not associated with death from stroke after multivariate adjustment. The results suggest inverse associations between death from stroke and intake of the most concentrated vitamin E food sources consumed by this cohort: mayonnaise, nuts, and margarine. These results suggest a protective effect of vitamin E from foods on death from stroke but do not support a protective role for supplemental vitamin E or other antioxidant vitamins; however, given the number of stroke deaths, a small-to-moderate association for the latter could not be ruled out (Yochum et al., 2000).

Another recent study examined the relationship between benign ovarian tumors (BOTs) and nutrients, primarily dietary fat, using case-control data (Britton, Westhoff, Howe, & Gammon, 2000). Six hundred and seventy-three cases and 351 controls provided dietary information. The risk of BOTs was elevated for those with the highest intake of total, vegetable, saturated, monounsaturated, and polyunsaturated fat. Elevated risks were observed for higher intakes of polyunsaturated fat with endometrioid, serous, and teratoma tumors. Higher intakes of vegetable fat, adjusted for polyunsaturated fat, increased the risk of endometrioid, mucinous, and serous tumors. Only the risk of serous BOTs was consistently lower for higher intakes of micronutrients, with the strongest reduction observed for sources of vitamin A. Findings were that polyunsaturated and vegetable fat may increase the risk of BOTs, while vitamin A may lower the risk of serous BOTs; however, these findings and lack of associations for other nutrients should be replicated (Britton et al., 2000).

BENEFITS OF EATING FISH

Mounting evidence about the cardiovascular benefits of fish led the American Heart Association to recommend eating two servings of fish a week. Eating fish, even in modest amounts, can significantly reduce a woman's risk of the most common type of stroke. A study of nearly 80,000 women found that eating fish was linked to reductions in the risk of ischemic, or clot-related, strokes, which account for about 83 percent of all strokes. Women who ate about 4 ounces of fish two to four times weekly cut their risk of ischemic stroke by 48 percent. Slightly higher risk reductions were found in women who ate fish five or more times weekly, but there were relatively few women in that group. Slight risk reductions were also found even in those who ate fish once a week or less (Iso et al., 2001). Omega-3 fatty acids, found in most fish, have been shown to lower levels of blood fats linked to cardiovascular disease and to help keep blood from clotting. The fats are especially plentiful in dark, oily fish such as mackerel, salmon, and sardines. While previous research largely has focused on fish and heart disease, the new study is one of the few to examine the effect on stroke risk and to differentiate between types of strokes.

Some researchers have suggested that eating large amounts of fish might increase the risk of hemorrhagic strokes, which occur when a blood vessel in the brain ruptures and bleeds. But one study found that a regular diet of fish neither increased nor decreased the risk of this type of stroke, which accounts for about one-fifth of all strokes. The researchers examined about 14 years of data on 79,839 participants in the Nurses' Health Study. The women were ages 34 to 59 in 1980. There were 574 strokes during the ensuing 14 years. The researchers took into account the women's age and whether they smoked, factors that could affect stroke risk. But other factors, such as high blood pressure, were not included.

POSSIBLE PROBLEMS OF EATING FISH

Fish is widely considered part of a healthy diet, but some types of fish can harbor high amounts of mercury, an element found naturally in the environment that is also a pollutant. There is recent evidence that some fish contain mercury levels toxic to humans, especially pregnant women. Two South American studies found contaminated fish in coastal waters. One survey was in the region of Alta Floresta in the south of the Amazon basin, close to the Teles Pires River. Women at different pregnancy stages were tested clinically and interviewed with a questionnaire. Mercury concentrations ranging from 0.05 to 8.2 were found among the women. Fish consumption was an important dietary protein source and also a possible exposure pathway, due to the high mercury concentrations reported in local carnivorous animal species (Hacon et al., 2000). Another study investigated exposure to methylmercury (MeHg) and mercury vapor (Hg0) in pregnant women and their newborns in Stockholm, Sweden. The women were followed for 15 months after delivery. Blood MeHg decreased during pregnancy, partly due to decreased intake of fish in accordance with recommendations to not eat certain predatory fish during pregnancy (Vahter et al., 2000).

In 2001 the U.S. Food and Drug Administration (FDA) released a statement that pregnant women and those who might become pregnant should not eat four types of fish—shark, swordfish, king mackerel, and tilefish—because they could contain enough mercury to hurt a fetus's developing brain.

WOMEN'S HEALTH AS A GLOBAL ISSUE

Women's health is a global issue. In developing countries, the health and nutrition of females throughout the life span is affected by complex and highly interrelated biological, social, cultural, and health service-related factors (Mora & Nestel, 2000). Rather than focusing exclusively on the prenatal period, health care providers will want to develop a life cycle approach to improving maternal nutrition, which goes beyond the traditional provision of nutrition services during pregnancy, by addressing risk factors that are present well before pregnancy, even before childbearing age. Policy actions and the components for effective implementation of such a program and the prospects and challenges to be overcome include:

- translating scientific knowledge into action, removing conceptual and implementational constraints.
- identifying biologically meaningful indicators for problem identification.
- improving understanding of physiological and social adaptation mechanisms as persistent problems within health care delivery systems.

Improving women's health and nutrition could save millions of women in developing countries from needless suffering or premature death. Cost-effective health interventions exist to prevent this loss of lives. Malnutrition is a major contributory factor to women's poor health and preventable mortality. Women's health is influenced by complex biological, social, and cultural factors that are highly interrelated. Significant progress can be achieved by strengthening and expanding an essential package of health services for women, improving the policy environment, and promoting more positive attitudes and behavior toward women's health (Tinker, 2000).

Men

Men have their own special nutrition needs. Increasing evidence links diet and lifestyle to health and illness. In general, men would do well to eat monounsaturated oils such as olive or canola oil. Vegetables, fruits, and soy products are rich in antioxidants that are essential to lower disease risk stemming from reactive oxygen systems in the body. Green and black teas are excellent sources of polyphenol antioxidants, as are cocoa and some chocolates (Weisburger, 2000).

DIET AND ITS PREVENTIVE ROLE IN PROSTATIC DISEASE

Asian men have much lower incidences of prostate cancer and possibly of benign prostatic hyperplasia (BPH) than their Western counterparts. Vegetarian men also have a lower incidence of prostate cancer than omnivorous males. Both Asian and vegetarian men consume low-fat, high-fiber diets that provide a rich supply of weak dietary oestrogens. These plants or phytoestrogens have been proposed as chemopreventive agents, particularly for Asian men, and to a lesser extent, for vegetarian men also. The three principal classes of phytoestrogens are the isoflavonoids, flavonoids, and lignans. Many foods of plant origin contain varying amounts of these compounds and hundreds of plants manifest some degree of oestrogenic activity. Soya, a dietary staple in many parts of Asia, is a major source of the isoflavonoids daidzein and genistein. Flavonoids are present in high concentration in many fruits, vegetables, and crop species. In particular, apigenin and kaempferol are regarded as major flavonoids because of their common occurrence in plants, and their significant concentrations when present. Apples, onions, and tea leaves are excellent sources of flavonoids. Plant lignans are present in many cereals, grains, fruits, and vegetables, and give rise to the mammalian lignans enterodiol and enterolactone; however, the richest source is linseed (flaxseed) and other oilseeds. In addition to their oestrogenic activity, many of these plant compounds can interfere with steroid metabolism and bioavailability, and also inhibit enzymes, such as tyrosine kinase and topoisomerase, which are crucial to cellular proliferation (Denis, Morton, & Griffiths, 1999).

One study found that men who reported low levels of physical activity had increased risk of prostate cancer compared with very active men. Lower levels of recreational activity were weakly associated with increased prostate cancer risk among African Americans but not among Caucasians. These results suggest that inactive men are at increased risk of prostate cancer (Clarke & Whittemore, 1999).

ALCOHOL AND PROSTATE CANCER

Researchers prospectively investigated the association between alcohol consumption and prostate cancer in the Epidemiologic Follow-up Study (NHEFS) of the first National Health and Nutrition Examination Survey (NHANES I). Alcohol consumption was assessed at baseline as usual consumption, and at follow-up as usual consumption and as distant past consumption at the ages of 25, 35, 45, and 55. There were 252 incident cases of prostate cancer. Consistent with most previous studies, there was no significant association between usual total alcohol consumption and prostate cancer, except for a significant inverse association at the heaviest level of drinking. Further study of heavy drinkers revealed significant inverse associations between distant past heavy drinking (defined as more than 25 drinks/week) and prostate cancer at age 25, age 35, and age 45, but not at age 55. These results suggest that it may be important to consider distant past alcohol consumption in etiologic studies of prostate cancer (Breslow et al., 1999).

HEALTHFUL EATING

Men are encouraged to eat a health-promoting daily diet including 5 to 10 servings of vegetables, fruits, and juices. Red wine and tea are rich sources of micronutrients with antioxidant properties, including the antioxidant vitamins C, E, and beta-carotene. However, it is important to limit intake of any wine to one to two drinks daily. Tomatoes contain lycopene, a stable, active antioxidant. Many vegetables contain quercetin and related polyphenolic compounds. Green tea is a source of epigallocatechin gallate, and black tea is a source of theaflavin and the associated thearubigins. Red wine contains resveratro (Weisburger, 2000). The diverse antioxidants in foods, red wine, and tea provide the necessary resources for the body to control oxidation reactions in the body with possible adverse consequences. For example, the oxidation of low density lipoprotein (LDL) cholesterol yields a product that damages the vascular system. Thus, a lower intake of saturated fats to decrease the levels of LDL cholesterol, together with an adequate intake of antioxidants, is the optimal approach to lower heart disease risk.

ELDERS

Demographics

The elderly population is the fastest growing segment in the United States today. One in seven Americans are over 65. The fastest growing segment of old people are those now classified as the "old-old," seniors over age 85. The challenge for us is to reach out to our burgeoning elderly population and guide them in the whys and wherefores of healing nutrition before they succumb to the preventable ravages of faulty nutrition.

Thanks to improved living conditions, better nutrition, preventive care, increased fitness, antibiotics, and other factors, more Americans will remain healthy through their 80s and beyond (Rapport, 2000). As people live longer, however, so too do their needs increase. Aging is associated with increased risk of developing anemia and micronutrient deficiencies (Olivares, Hertrampf, Capurro, & Wegner, 2000).

CASE STUDY: Mike

Mike, an 87-year-old retired executive, lived in an exclusive apartment building in an elite section of a major city. The widower had two daughters, aged 60 and 64, who lived with their children in an adjoining state and seldom visited, and a successful son nearing retirement in a distant state. Mike had an income of $2,600 a month and a quarter of a million dollars in assets, yet he was starving to death. Neither his remaining few friends nor his relatives realized he was subsisting on over-the-counter coffee cakes and root beers.

Mike arose each day at 6:00 A.M., brewed a pot of coffee, and lounged through the morning reading the paper and working on his investment accounts. In the late morning, he went out to a local café and ordered the breakfast pastry of the day, usually a wedge of high-fat, high-sugar coffee cake. On most days, he had another cup of coffee to wash down the pastry

(Continued on next page)

and then strolled through the park and neighborhood, making his way home around 1:00 P.M.

He knew that a local senior center offered midday meals, but he had a prejudice against that group. He thought only low-income people went there. Also, he had become quite antisocial since the death of his wife two years ago. During the afternoon, he tinkered with model cars, a hobby he had never had time for during his working years. More often than not, he took a nap during the afternoon. When he awoke, he liked to have a frosty root beer. He kept a good stock in his kitchen. At 6:00 P.M., he turned on the television and usually flipped channels and watched programs while he resumed work on his model cars and drank from his stock of root beer.

On weekends, one of his children would call or he would call them. On holidays, he usually traveled to one of their homes and stayed a night or two. He ate sparsely because his stomach had shrunk and his appetite waned. No one particularly noticed, and no changes occurred. It was not until two years later, when a much older, feeble Mike fell and sprained his ankle that anyone paid any attention to his health.

At the emergency department of the city hospital, the staff decided to admit Mike for observation. An intake assessment revealed that Mike was suffering from malnutrition related to inadequate nutrition. Skin lesions, emaciation, and muscle wasting were among the overt external signs. The internal changes would also have to be assessed and corrected. Both would require time, effort, money, and reeducation.

Observation

Mike is representative of millions of older adults. As the 21st century progresses, there are going to be increasing numbers of people like Mike— elders who, while trying to adjust to the changes of old age, forget the importance of eating. Economic status is not a factor in geriatric malnutrition; it can happen to any elder left alone. Gerontology offers an area of specialization that is becoming increasingly meaningful with the growing number of people who need health care practitioners to guide them into a graceful, fulfilling, healthy old age.

Nutrition Facts for Older Adults

Energy expenditure and caloric intake typically decline with age. As nutrient and caloric intake decline, a parallel decline in vitamin and mineral intake is inevitable. A contributing factor is that many elderly people live alone and often do not bother to cook for themselves. The result is that many mature adults do not enjoy food as much as they did. Many must literally make themselves sit down and eat meals. Consequently, they tend to eat more comfort foods, such as puddings, cakes, and cookies. Unfortunately sweet foods do not provide the nutrients they need.

Many elderly people have trouble eating or swallowing because of tooth pain or ill-fitting dentures. Many live on low or fixed incomes, and some take medications that cause adverse nutrient interactions. Their appetites may be reduced, their senses of taste and smell may be impaired, or they may suffer from chronic diseases. All of these factors contribute to the declining nutritional status of our valuable senior citizens. By increasing our awareness of these facts and by recognizing that increasing numbers of people like Mike will be needing nursing services, we will be in a better position to discover ways to better serve this population.

Overweight, drinking and driving, inadequate fruit and vegetable consumption, physical inactivity, and smoking are associated with the leading causes of morbidity and mortality among people over 65 years in the United States (Kamimoto, Easton, Maurice, Husten, & Macera, 1999). Data from the Behavioral Risk Factor Surveillance System (BRFSS) for 1994–1997 and from the National Health Interview Survey (NHIS) for 1993–1995 have been used for surveillance purposes. With education and attention, prevalence of overweight, drinking and driving, inadequate fruit and vegetable consumption, and smoking decrease with increasing age; physical inactivity is the primary health risk that increases with increasing age. Specific subgroups of older adults are at risk, and these health risks vary by age, race, residential state, and socioeconomic status and highlight the heterogeneous nature of older adults. Surveillance for health risks among older adults provides information to help identify effective interventions for the growing population of older adults in the United States (Kamimoto et al., 1999).

In one recent study a nutritional assessment of low-income, elderly African Americans was undertaken to develop appropriate nutritional intervention programs suitable for their needs and tastes to ensure maximum compliance. Twenty-three subjects (18 women and 5 men) 60 to 82 years old participated in the study. A majority of the subjects had an income of $5,000 to $10,000 per year and an education level below junior high school. Eighteen subjects had hypertension and eight of those also had diabetes mellitus. Weights ranged from 131 to 265 pounds, and blood cholesterol levels varied from 200 to 288 mg/dl. Their diets were high in sodium and fat and low in fresh fruits and vegetables. Based on this preliminary information, an instrument to assess the nutritional knowledge of this population and a nutrition education program are being developed to aid in developing nutrition education modules for the low-income elderly African American population in the United States (Kaul & Nidiry, 2000).

The prevalence of malnutrition, which is relatively low in free-living elderly persons (5 to 10 percent), is considerably higher (30 to 60 percent) in hospitalized or institutionalized elderly persons (Vellas et al., 2001). Hospital stay is often associated with further weight loss (Potter, 2001). As a result, nutritional assessment should be part of routine clinical practice in elderly patients who are frail, sick, or hospitalized. A comprehensive screening tool for assessment of nutritional status that is clinically relevant and cost-effective to perform is needed. A number of simple and rapid tests for detecting or diagnosing malnutrition in the elderly have recently been developed. If malnutrition is suggested by such screening tests, then they should be supplemented by conventional nutritional assessment before treatment is planned (Vellas et al., 2001).

SUMMARY

Our bodies are constantly changing. Our 400 billion cells develop, grow, die, and are shed continuously. During active stages of life we need micronutrients and calories in greater quanties than during other, more quiescent stages of life. There are different needs and different requirements for men and women. In the 21st century, much greater emphasis will be focused on maximizing the health of adult men and women who were previously understudied. Just as we learn what best to do, we also learn what we should not do or not eat. All health care providers should be aware of needs during various stages during the life span so that we can better assist people as they heal and evolve through better nutrition.

REFERENCES

Breslow, R. A., Wideroff, L., Graubard, B. I., Erwin, D., Reichman, M. E., Ziegler, R. G., & Ballard-Barbash, R. (1999). Alcohol and prostate cancer in the NHANES I epidemiologic follow-up study. First National Health and Nutrition Examination Survey of the United States. *Annals of Epidemiology, 9*(4), 254–261.

Britton, J. A., Westhoff, C., Howe, G., & Gammon, M. D. (2000). Diet and benign ovarian tumors (United States). *Cancer Causes Control, 11*(5), 389–401.

Choay, P. (2000). Micronutritional requirements during women's life. *Annales Pharmaceutiques Francaises, 58*(6 Suppl.), 443–447.

Clarke, G., & Whittemore, A. S. (2000). Prostate cancer risk in relation to anthropometry and physical activity: The National Health and Nutrition Examination Survey I Epidemiological Follow-Up Study. *Cancer Epidemiological Biomarkers Prevalence, 9*(9), 875–881.

Denis, L., Morton, M. S., & Griffiths, K. (1999). Diet and its preventive role in prostatic disease. *Euoropean Urology, 35*(5–6), 377–387.

Giardina, E. G. (2000). Heart disease in women. *International Journal of Fertility and Womens Medicine, 45*(6), 350–357.

Hacon, S., Yokoo, E., Valente, J., Campos, R. C., da Silva, V. A., de Menezes, A. C., de Moraes, L. P., & Ignotti, E. (2000). Exposure to mercury in pregnant women from Alta Floresta-Amazon Basin, Brazil. *Environmental Research, 84*(3), 204–210.

Hass, E. (2000). Programs for childhood. In *Staying healthy with nutrition: The complete guide to diet and nutrition.* Boston: Celestial Arts.

Iso, H., Reprode, K. M., Stanpfer, M. J., Manson, J. E., Colditz, G. A., Speizer, F. E., Hennekens, C. H., & Willett, W. C. (2001). Intake of fish and omega-3 fatty acids and risk of stroke in women. *JAMA, 285*(3), 304–312.

Kaluski, D. N., & Levental, A. (1999). Nutrition for women's health. *Harefuah, 137*(12), 606–609, 679.

Kaminoto, L. A., Easton, A. N., Maurice, E., Husten, C. G., & Macera, C. A. (1999). Surveillance for five health risks among older adults—United States 1993–1997. Morbidity and Mortality weekly report. CDC surveillance summaries, 48(8), 51–88.

Kaul, L., & Nidiry, J. J. (2000). Nutritional assessment of low-income elderly African-American population. *Journal of the National Medical Association, 92*(11), 524–527.

King, K. B., & Mosca, L. (2000). Prevention of heart disease in women: Recommendations for management of risk factors. *Progress in Cardiovascular Nursing, 15*(2), 36–42.

La Croix, A. Z., Newton, K. M., Leveille, S. G., & Wallace, J. (1997). Healthy aging. A women's issue. *Western Journal of Medicine, 167*(4), 220–232.

Lindsay, S. H., & Claywell, L. G. (1999). Considering soy: Its estrogenic effects may protect women. *Journal of Obstetrics and Gynecology Neonatal Nursing, 28*(6 Suppl. 1), 21–24.

Liu, S., Manson, J. E., Lee, I. M., Cole, S. R., Hennekens, C. H., Willett, W. C., & Buring, J. E. (2000). Fruit and vegetable intake and risk of cardiovascular disease: The Women's Health Study. *American Journal of Clinical Nutrition, 72*(4), 922–928.

McGowan, J. A., & Pottern, L. (2000). Commentary on the Women's Health Initiative. *Maturitas, 34*(2), 109–112.

Mora, J. O., & Nestel, P. S. (2000). Improving prenatal nutrition in developing countries: Strategies, prospects, and challenges. *American Journal of Clinical Nutrition, 71*(5 Suppl.), 1353S–1363S.

Olivares, M., Hertrampf, E., Capurro, M. T., & Wegner, D. (2000). Prevalence of anemia in elderly subjects living at home: Role of micronutrient deficiency and inflammation. *European Journal of Clinical Nutrition, 54*(11), 834–839.

Potter, J. M. (2001). Oral supplements in the elderly. *Current Opinions in Clinical Nutrition and Metabolic Care, 4*(1), 21–28.

Rapport, R. (2000). Senior health issues. *New England Journal of Medicine, 97*(6), 43–44.

Thorand, B., Kohlmcicr, L., Simonscn, N., Croghan, C., & Thamm, M. (1998). Intake of fruits, vegetables, folic acid, and related nutrients and risk of breast cancer in postmenopausal women. *Public Health Nutrition, 1*(3), 147–156.

Tinker, A. (2000). Women's health: The unfinished agenda. *International Journal of Gynaecology and Obstetrics, 70*(1), 149–158.

Vahter, M., Akesson, A., Lind, B., Bjors, U., Schutz, A., & Berglund, M. (2000). Longitudinal study of methylmercury and inorganic mercury in blood and urine of pregnant and lactating women, as well as in umbilical cord blood. *Environmental Research, 84*(2), 186–194.

Vellas, B., Lauque, S., Andrieu, S., Nourhashemi, F., Rolland, Y., Baumgartner, R., & Garry, P. (2001). Nutrition assessment in the elderly. *Current Opinions in Clinical Nutrition and Metabolic Care, 4*(1), 5–8.

Weisburger, J. H. (2000). Mechanisms of action of antioxidants as exemplified in vegetables, tomatoes, and tea. *Food and Chemical Toxicology, 37*(9–10), 943–948.

Yochum, L. A., Folsom, A. R., & Kushi, L. H. (2000). Intake of antioxidant vitamins and risk of death from stroke in postmenopausal women. *American Journal of Clinical Nutrition, 72*(2), 476–483.

PART III

New Dimensions
of Healing
Foods

CHAPTER 11

New Food Facts

FOOD LABELING

New food labeling laws went into effect in 1994. Prior to this consumer legislation, the nutritional content of processed foods was a mystery to grocery store customers. Food products must now carry generic labels so that shoppers can make informed choices when selecting foods from supermarket shelves. Generally, all processed food items must display a label detailing selected nutritional facts. The label begins with serving size and number of servings per container, followed by amount of calories per serving, including how many of these calories come from fat. The next area lists total fat, cholesterol, sodium, a breakdown of carbohydrates, and protein. The percentages of vitamins and minerals follow.

Foods Not Covered

Not every food item is required to carry the new label. Raw, single-ingredient meat and poultry products, fresh fish, and 20 of the most popular fruits and vegetables do not have to comply. Other exempt items include foods served in restaurants, purchased in delicatessens, sold in small packages, or produced by small businesses. Other exceptions to the nutritional panel format are allowed on labels of foods made specifically for children under the age of 4 because the FDA has not established daily values for this age group.

Reading the Label

The new food labels can contribute greatly to savvy shoppers' diets. By carefully reading and comparing labels, consumers can make healthy choices in food selection. For example, when comparing labels you might be surprised to learn that a can of soup has 35 calories of fat per serving, while a serving of baked snack chips has only 30 calories from fat. On the same label, we read that the soup has 7 percent of the daily value of cholesterol, while the snack chips have no cholesterol. If you have not yet begun the practice of label reading, start now. You will be amazed at the difference it can make in controlling your nutrient intake. Figure 11–1 shows a Nutrition Facts label.

Legal Labeling

The Federal Drug Administration (FDA) recognizes different categories of foods, one of which is foods in conventional food form, the most prevalent foods in the general food supply. Within the conventional food group is a group called *foods for special dietary use* (FSDU). The term *special dietary use* as applied to food means particular (as distinguished from general) uses of food that fulfill a dietary need which exists by reason of a physical, physiologic, pathologic, or other condition including, but not limited to, diseases, convalescence, pregnancy, lactation, allergen hypersensitivity, underweight, or overweight. Both conventional foods and FSDU are subject to the labeling requirements of the Nutrition Labeling and

Nutrition Facts

Serving Size 1/2 cup (114 g)
Servings per container 4

Amount per Serving

Calories 90	Calories from Fat 30

	% Daily Value*
Total Fat 3g	5%
Saturated Fat 0g	0%
Cholesterol 0mg	0%
Sodium 300mg	13%
Total Carbohydrate 13g	4%
Dietary Fiber 3g	12%
Sugars 3g	
Protein 3g	

Vitamin A	80%	•	Vitamin C	60%
Calcium	4%	•	Iron	4%

*Percent Daily Values are based on a 2,000 calorie diet. Your daily values may be higher or lower depending on your calorie needs:

	Calories	2,000	2,500
Total Fat	Less than	65g	80g
Sat Fat	Less than	20 mg	25 mg
Cholesterol	Less than	300 mg	300mg
Sodium	Less than	2,400mg	2,400mg
Total Carbohydrate		300g	375g
Fiber		25g	30g

Calories per gram:
Fat 9 • Carbohydrates 4 • Protein 4

Figure 11–1 The Nutrition Facts food label.
Source: Food and Drug Administration, 1992.

Education Act (NLEA) of 1990, as well as the general food safety requirements. The only substances that may be used in foods are food ingredients whose use is safe and suitable under the applicable food safety provisions; that is, the substance is generally recognized as safe (GRAS) for such use, is used in accordance with the FDA's food additive regulations, or is authorized by a prior sanction. In addition, regulations require that the food be a safe, clean, and wholesome product and that its labeling be truthful and not misleading (Ross, 2000).

Foods may be classified into a range of legal and regulatory categories. This gives manufacturers and retailers who wish to develop functional foods a great deal of flexibility. The primary determinant of the regulatory status of a food is its intended use, which is largely reflected by the label and by labeling information accompanying the product. The labeling provisions enumerated under the NLEA, and implemented by FDA regulations as mandated in the Code of Federal Regulations, specify that labels provide the nutrient composition or nutrient facts of a food product. Several nutrients (e.g., vitamins A and C) must be declared when they are in the product. Declaration of certain other nutrients on the label is optional. Declarations must state the amount per serving and as a percentage of the daily value. In 1997, the FDA published final rules governing the nutrition labeling of dietary supplements; these regulations became effective in 1999 (Ross, 2000).

Other mandatory information for food labels includes a statement of identity (common or usual name of the product); an accurate statement of the net quantity of contents; the name and place of the business, manufacturer, packer, or distributor; and, if the food was fabricated from two or more ingredients, a complete list of those ingredients, in descending order of predominance, by their common or usual names. All labeling information must appear in English. In addition, if a label bears any representation in a foreign language, all mandatory label information must be repeated in that language. These regulations also apply to dietary supplements.

Health claims can also be made on food labels. Under the NLEA, once authorized by regulation, these claims may be used on any food and dietary supplement that meets the qualifying criteria for amount of nutrient per serving and other requirements. A petition process is available for seeking FDA authorization for new claims. New provisions for making both health and nutrient content claims were included in the Food and Drug Administration Modernization Act of 1997. Health claim messages must reference both the food substance and outcomes related to disease or health. The science standard to support the claim of a relationship between a food substance and disease or health must be based on the totality of publicly available scientific evidence (Ross, 2000).

The FDA conducts studies of food labels as part of its ongoing monitoring of the nutritional status of the U.S. population. In 2000, three years after implementation of the final nutrition labeling rules in 1997, labeled products accounted for an estimated 96.5 percent of the annual sales of processed, packaged foods.

An additional 3.4 percent of products sold were exempt from labeling regulations. Nutrient content claims and health claims appeared on an estimated 39 percent and 4 percent, respectively, of the products sold. Dietitians and other health care professionals can use this information to identify food types with specific label information and to assist clients in making more varied and healthful food choices in the marketplace (Brecher, Bender, Wilkening, McCabe, & Anderson, 2000).

Current Research

One recent research study measured the reported use of nutrition information on food labels by a population of university students to determine if label users differed from nonusers in terms of gender and specific beliefs related to label information and diet-disease relationships, specifically fat and heart disease and fiber and cancer. A total of 553 students in randomly selected classes took part in the survey. The sample consisted of roughly equal numbers of males and females, between the ages of 18 and 24. There were approximately equal numbers of label users and nonusers among males, while label users outnumbered nonusers by almost four to one among females. It seems that females use food labels more often than do males. The importance of nutrition information on food labels was the only belief that differed significantly between label users and nonusers for both sexes. For females, no other beliefs distinguished label users from nonusers. However, for males, significant differences were found between label users and nonusers regarding the beliefs that nutrition information is truthful and that a relationship between fiber and cancer exists. The only consistently observed difference between label users and nonusers (male and female) was that users believed in the importance of nutrition information on food labels while nonusers did not (Smith, Taylor, & Stephen, 2000).

Another study evaluated awareness and use of a supermarket-shelf labeling program designed to encourage shoppers to make food choices that promote heart health. The shelf-labeling program was implemented in 18 supermarkets serving minority communities in Detroit, Michigan. Customers were given an exit survey to determine awareness and use of the program. Of the 361-person sample, 66 percent were female, 67 percent were African American, and the sample population had a mean age of 51 years. Overall awareness of the program was a modest 28.8 percent, though awareness of the program among minorities was significantly higher than compared with whites (35.3 percent versus 20.8 percent). Gender, age, and education level were not predictive of program awareness but people screened for cardiovascular disease risk factors (elevated low-density lipoprotein or total cholesterol levels and/or elevated blood pressure) in the previous year had greater awareness than those who had not been screened. Among subjects aware of the program, 56 percent actually used it, a figure that did not differ significantly by gender, age, or ethnicity. This finding suggests that shelf labels have the potential to increase the selection of foods that promote heart health in predominately low-income, minority populations (Lang, Mercer, Tran, & Mosca, 2000).

THE FOOD PYRAMID

Most health care providers know about the pyramid conceptualized by Abraham Maslow in his theory of the hierarchy of human needs. The principle in Maslow's pyramid is that we need to meet basic physiologic needs before advancing to the apex of self-actualization. Since the pyramid concept is easy to grasp, food theorists have devised their own food guide pyramid. This pyramid is a general guide that outlines what we need to eat each day to maintain basic requirements. The illustrations of the four food groups and the food group wheel that were used in general and professional education for so long are obsolete. In April of 1992, the U.S. Department of Agriculture (USDA), with the endorsement of the U.S. Department of Health and Human Services (DHHS) issued the Food Guide Pyramid to illustrate the new food categories.

At the base of the pyramid are foods that come from grains. The bulk of our dietary intake should come from this area. These foods supply fiber, complex carbohydrates, vitamins, and minerals. The second level represents fruits and vegetables. Foods from plants supply multiple and diverse nutrient needs. The third level includes meat, poultry, fish, dry beans, eggs, and nuts. These are important sources of protein, iron, and zinc. Adjacent to this group is the milk, yogurt, and cheese group. Calcium and protein are the primary nutrients in this group. Vegetables and fruits are more necessary than protein foods. The small tip of the pyramid represents fats, oils, and sweets. This group includes salad dressings, oils, butter, margarine, cream, soft drinks, candy, and sweet desserts. These foods provide calories but little else nutritionally. Figure 11–2 depicts the Food Guide Pyramid.

One of the hallmarks of the food pyramid guide is that it is based on a recommended number of servings for each of the levels on the pyramid. Serving sizes are shown in Table 11–1. If you eat a larger portion, it gets counted as an additional serving. For example, ½ cup of cooked pasta counts as one serving in the bread group. If you eat 1 cup of pasta, that counts as 2 servings. If you eat a smaller portion, count it as part of a serving. Use servings as a general guide. For mixed foods, estimate the food group serving of the main ingredients. For example, a large slice of pizza counts in the bread group (crust), the milk group (cheese), and the vegetable group (tomato sauce). A cup-size helping of beef stew counts as one serving of meat and one serving of vegetables.

Table 11–2 gives samples of how many servings from each group are recommended for each of the calorie categories. The calorie category allocations are discussed in Chapter 4, Basic Nutritional Needs.

Food Guide Pyramid
A Guide to Daily Food Choices

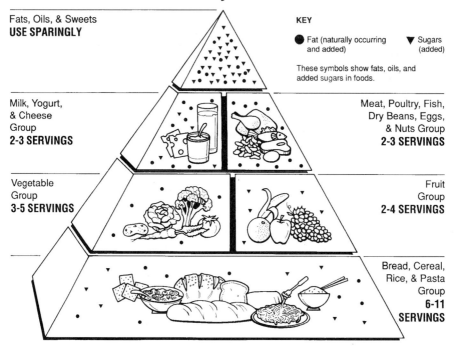

Fats, Oils, & Sweets
USE SPARINGLY

KEY

● Fat (naturally occurring and added) ▼ Sugars (added)

These symbols show fats, oils, and added sugars in foods.

Milk, Yogurt, & Cheese Group
2-3 SERVINGS

Meat, Poultry, Fish, Dry Beans, Eggs, & Nuts Group
2-3 SERVINGS

Vegetable Group
3-5 SERVINGS

Fruit Group
2-4 SERVINGS

Bread, Cereal, Rice, & Pasta Group
6-11 SERVINGS

Figure 11–2 The Food Guide Pyramid.
Source: U.S. Department of Agriculture and the U.S. Department of Health and Human Services. Provided by the Education Department of the National Live Stock and Meat Board.

The food pyramid is easy to understand and follow. Instead of thinking of foods in four groups, reorient your thinking to pyramids.

THE MEDITERRANEAN DIET PYRAMID

The most recent and still controversial nutrition plan to emerge is the Mediterranean Diet Pyramid. The Mediterranean diet proposal was created by a team of nutritionists and epidemiologists from the World Health Organization (WHO) and Harvard's School of Public Health. The team spent two years devising this new plan as a response to the USDA Food Guide Pyramid. Their goal was to emulate those parts of the Mediterranean region that in the recent past have enjoyed the lowest recorded rates of chronic disease and the highest adult life expectancy. The proposal features its own pyramid along with recommendations

TABLE 11–1 Food Serving Sizes

FOOD ITEM	AMOUNT IN SERVING
Bread, cereal, rice, pasta	1 oz. ready-to-eat cereal ½ cup cooked cereal, rice, or pasta 1 slice of bread ½ bagel or hamburger bun
Vegetable	1 cup raw, leafy vegetables ½ cup other vegetables, cooked or raw ¾ cup of vegetable juice
Fruit	½ cup of cooked or canned fruit 1 medium apple, banana, or orange ¾ cup of fruit juice
Milk, yogurt, or cheese	1 cup milk or yogurt 1½ oz. natural cheese 2 oz. processed cheese
Meat, poultry, fish, beans, eggs, and nuts	½ cup cooked dry beans 1 egg 2–3 oz. cooked lean meat, poultry, or fish 4 tbsp. peanut butter

for consuming one or two glasses of wine a day and engaging in physical activity (see Figure 11–3 on page 144).

The call for the daily dose of wine, as shown with an asterisk at the base of the figure, adds new heat to one of the biggest controversies in public health today. Growing evidence suggests that wine plays a role in protecting against heart

TABLE 11–2 Suggested Daily Servings Based on Caloric Needs

FOOD GROUP	1,600 CALORIES	2,200 CALORIES	2,800 CALORIES
Bread group servings	6	9	11
Vegetable group servings	3	4	5
Fruit group servings	2	3	4
Milk group servings	2–3*	2–3*	2–3*
Meat group (in ounces)	5**	6**	7*
Total fat (in grams)	53	73	93
Added sugars (in tsp.)+	6	12	18

**Young adults 18 to 24 years old need 3 servings. Teenagers 11 to 18 years and pregnant women need 4 servings. Lactating women need 5 servings.
**Pregnant women need 6 ounces of meat per day and lactating women need 7 to 8 ounces of meat per day.
+Added from candy, desserts, soft drinks, and other sweets.

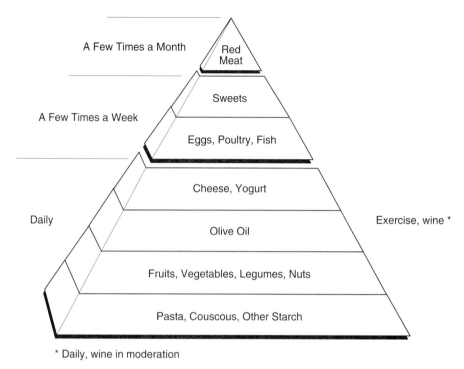

A Few Times a Month — Red Meat

A Few Times a Week — Sweets; Eggs, Poultry, Fish

Cheese, Yogurt

Daily — Olive Oil — **Exercise, wine ***

Fruits, Vegetables, Legumes, Nuts

Pasta, Couscous, Other Starch

* Daily, wine in moderation

Figure 11–3 Mediterranean Diet Pyramid.

disease, but only when consumed in moderation. The problem, of course, is that many people use more than recommended. Thus, from a contemporary public health perspective, wine should be considered optional.

Current Research

Low mortality in Mediterranean populations has stimulated much interest, with researchers citing diet as the most likely explanation. A prospective cohort study, involving 141 Anglo-Celts and 189 Greek-Australians of both sexes 70 years or older, was done in Australia to evaluate whether adherence to the Mediterranean diet affects survival of elderly people in developed non-Mediterranean countries. Diet was assessed using an extensive validated questionnaire on food intake. A one unit increase in a diet score based on eight key features of the traditional common diet in the Mediterranean region was associated with a 17 percent reduction in overall mortality. Mortality reduction with increasing diet score was at least as evident among Anglo-Celts as among Greek-Australians. The researchers concluded that a diet that adheres to the principles of the traditional Mediterranean diet is associated with longer survival among Australians of either Greek or Anglo-Celtic origin (Kouris-Blazos et al., 1999).

Another study analyzed data from Albania, the poorest country in Europe, to see if the situation there corroborates findings from elsewhere in the Mediterranean region. Demographic and food consumption data from United Nations agency sources were used to identify potential explanations for Albania's mortality pattern. Consistent with its economic situation, Albania has one of the highest infant mortality rates in Europe (45.4 per 1,000 live births for males and 38.0 for females in 1990). By contrast, adult mortality, including death from cardiovascular diseases, is similar to that in other Mediterranean countries. For example, age-standardized death from coronary heart disease in males to age 64 was 41 per 100,000 in Albania in 1990, less than half the rate in the United Kingdom but similar to that in Italy. Analysis of the geographical distribution of mortality within Albania (1978) showed that death rates were lowest in the southwest where most of the olive oil, fruits, and vegetables are produced and consumed. This paradox of high adult life expectancy in an extremely low-income country can be most plausibly explained by diet—namely, low consumption of total energy, meat, and milk products coupled with high consumption of fruit, vegetables, and carbohydrates (Gjonca & Bobak, 1997).

THE MEXICAN AMERICAN FOOD GUIDE PYRAMID

Mexican Americans make up a large segment of the U.S. population. Mexican food, increasing popular with everyone, is a combination of Spanish and Native American food. Beans, rice, chili peppers, tomatoes, and corn meal constitute a large part of the diet. Meat is often cooked with a sparse assortment of vegetables while corn meal or flour is used to make tortillas, which serve as the bread portion of meals. This diet is often limited in green and yellow vegetables and vitamin C–rich foods (Townsend & Roth, 2000). Those eating the Mexican American diet would be wise to add more greens such as spinach, salads, broccoli, brussel sprouts, and green beans. Figure 11–4 depicts the Mexican American diet in terms of a food pyramid.

SUMMARY

Within the past few years, we have witnessed dramatic changes in the organization and description of approaches to healthy eating. The Food Pyramid, the Mediterranean Diet Pyramid, and the Mexican American Food Guide Pyramid detail new dietary recommendations for the U.S. public, while new food labels guide us in selecting individual food products. When following the pyramid approaches, we will eat less meaty protein and increase fruits, grains, and complex carbohydrates. Some of us may prefer to choose the Mediterranean diet regime and include more olive oils and a daily glass of wine.

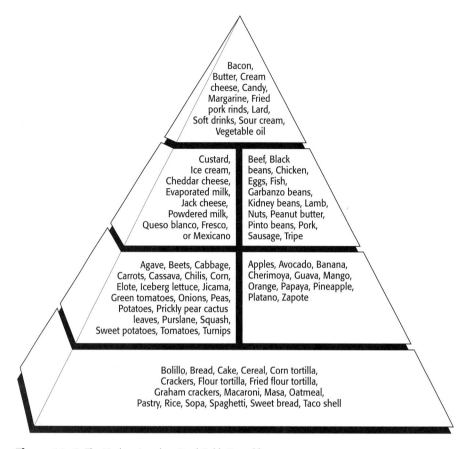

Figure 11–4 The Mexican American Food Guide Pyramid.
(© 1993 *Pyramid Packet* Penn State Nutrition Center, 417 East Calder Way, University Park, PA 16801-5633; 814-865-6323)

REFERENCES

Brecher, S. J., Bender, M. M., Wilkening, V. L., McCabe, N. M., & Anderson, E. M. (2000). Status of nutrition labeling, health claims, and nutrient content claims for processed foods: 1997 Food Label and Package Survey. *Journal of the American Dietetic Association, 100*(9), 1057–1062.

Gjonca, A., & Bobak, M. (1997). Albanian paradox, another example of protective effect of Mediterranean lifestyle? *Lancet, 350*(9094), 1815–1817.

Kouris-Blazos, A., Gnardellis, C., Wahlqvist, M. L., Trichopoulos, D., Lukito, W., & Trichopoulou, A. (1999). Are the advantages of the Mediterranean diet transferable to other populations? A cohort study in Melbourne, Australia. *British Journal of Nutrition, 82*(1), 57–61.

Lang, J. E., Mercer, N., Tran, D., & Mosca, L. (2000). Use of a supermarket shelf–labeling program to educate a predominately minority community about foods that promote heart health. *Journal of the American Dietetic Association, 100*(7), 804–809.

Ross, S. (2000). Functional foods: The Food and Drug Administration perspective. *American Journal of Clinical Nutrition, 71*(6 Suppl.), 1735S–1738S; discussion 1739S–1742S.

Smith, S. C., Taylor, J. G., & Stephen, A. M. (2000). Use of food labels and beliefs about diet-disease relationships among university students. *Public Health Nutrition, 3*(2), 175–182.

Townsend, C. E., & Roth, R. A. (2000). *Nutrition and Diet Therapy.* Albany, NY: Delmar.

CHAPTER 12

Living Foods

Some nutritionists believe that the closer food is to its living state, the better. The primary reason for this is that living foods contain living enzymes, which are the building blocks of cells. Most foods, despite their freshness, have been separated from their earth source and hence have begun the decaying process. Although it may be days, weeks, or in some cases months before the food deteriorates completely, nutrients begin the fading process immediately following harvest. The longer the time span from the reaping stage to the consumption stage, the greater the deterioration. Also, the greater the degree of processing the greater the amount of nutrient loss.

Some foods are still in a living state when we consume them. Yogurt and sprouted seeds are among the foods available to us in the living state. Salads and dishes made from fresh fruits and vegetables are the best known living foods.

SPROUTED SEEDS

The art of sprouting seeds is as old as recorded history. The use of sprouts was recorded in China as long ago as 2939 B.C.E. For a millennium, the majority of human foods came from grain seeds. Rice, millet, barley, oats, corn, sorghum, and rye have been staples around the globe throughout history. Legume seeds are also primary food sources. Lentils, dried beans, dried peas, and soybeans are rich in protein and carbohydrates. Other sources of seed foods are nuts such as almonds and walnuts.

Sprouted seeds have the reputation of power, which they get through the period of germination. Germination is the resumption of growth of a plant seed, spore, or bud after a period of dormancy. The main feature of germination is the increased rate of respiration, which is the biological "burning," or oxidation, of carbohydrates to provide energy for metabolism and growth. The viability, or the ability to germinate after prolonged periods of time, varies greatly among different species. Seeds are potent after they have germinated into sprouts. That is when we eat them. The most popular seeds used for sprouting are alfalfa, mung beans, chickpeas, and lentils.

In the West, sprouts were virtually unheard of a decade or two ago. Today, they are widely used in American cuisine in salads, as a replacement for lettuce on sandwiches, and in Chinese dishes.

Possible Health Hazards

There have been documented outbreaks of bacterial contamination associated with sprouts. Sprouts present a special problem because of the potential for pathogen growth during the sprouting process. If pathogens are present on or in the seed, sprouting conditions may favor their proliferation. There is no inherent step in the production of raw sprouts to reduce or eliminate pathogens. Contaminated seed is the likely source for most reported sprout-associated outbreaks. Research on methods to reduce or eliminate pathogenic bacteria on seeds and sprouts and some treatments show promise. However, to date, no single treatment has been shown to completely eliminate pathogens under experimental conditions used (National Advisory Committee, 1999).

Since there does not seem to be a way to completely eliminate the pathogens potential from sprouts, this has precipitated a review of current industry practices and initiatives related to the growing of seed and the production of sprouts. In 1997 the National Advisory Committee on Microbiological Criteria for Foods (NACMCF) reviewed the current literature on sprout-associated outbreaks to identify the organisms and production practices of greatest public health concern, prioritize research needs, and provide recommendations on intervention and prevention strategies. The committee's Fresh Produce Work Group (FPWG) found that there was a lack of fundamental food safety knowledge along the continuum from seed production through sprout consumption. Although seed appears to be the most likely source of contamination in sprout-associated outbreaks, practices and conditions at sprouting facilities may also affect the safety of the finished product. In recent sprout-associated outbreak investigations, facilities associated with outbreaks did not consistently apply seed disinfection treatments prior to sprouting. Notably, facilities that used seed from the same lots as implicated facilities, but were not associated with reported illnesses, appear to have consistently used seed disinfection treatments, such as 20,000 ppm calcium hypochlorite, to disinfect seed prior to sprouting. Out of NACMCF's work, a number of specific recommendations emerged (National Advisory Committee, 1999):

1. The knowledge of all interested parties pertaining to the microbiological safety of sprouted seeds must be enhanced; government and industry should develop education programs for seed and sprout producers on basic principles for microbiological food safety, good agricultural practices, good manufacturing practices, and hazard analysis and critical control point (HACCP) systems.

2. Good agricultural practices should be systematically implemented to reduce the potential for microbial contamination of seeds for sprout production.

3. Seed cleaning, storage, and handling practices that minimize the potential for microbial contamination should be developed and implemented.

4. Seeds should be treated with one or more treatments that have been shown to reduce pathogenic bacteria which may be present. Intervention strategies that deliver less than a specified reduction in levels of *Salmonella spp.* and enterohemorrhagic *Escherichia coli* O157 should be coupled with a microbiological testing program.

5. Good manufacturing practices and food safety systems, including regulatory oversight, microbial testing, adoption of HACCP, and improved traceback, that systematically look for means to prevent seeds from serving as the vehicle for food-borne disease should be established.

6. Research related to the microbiological safety of sprouted seeds, particularly in the areas of pathogen reduction or elimination, sources of contamination and its prevention, and preventing or retarding pathogen growth during sprouting, should be conducted.

Other investigators found naturally contaminated alfalfa seeds, epidemiologically linked to food-borne disease outbreaks in Oregon and British Columbia, and tested them for the presence of salmonella. Ten sample units from a suspected lot were sprouted and grown for 4 days. After enrichment of the grown sprouts, an enzyme immunoassay (EIA) and culture method were used to detect and isolate salmonella. Four of the 10 sample units were positive with the EIA; however, 5 of the 10 sample units were culture positive. The positive alfalfa seed sample units were further tested after shredding, soaking, and washing before culturing. Results suggest that sprouting and shredding methods may yield greater detection and recovery rates of salmonella (Inami & Moler, 1999).

YOGURT

Yogurt, a fermented, slightly acidic food product, is made from milk. Its origins are unknown, although the name comes from the Turkish language. Yogurt resembles many other fermented milk foods made throughout the world, such as kefir and kumiss. Unlike many of these foods, however, yogurt is usually made from a concentrated milk and is soured by a specific bacillus, *Lactobacillus bulgaricus*.

During the late 19th century, Elie Metchnikoff, a Russian biologist who worked in the Pasteur Institute in Paris, put forward the theory that the deterioration of the body was largely influenced by putrefactive bacteria that produced toxins in the large intestine. Noting the health and longevity of certain Balkan tribes for whom yogurt was a food staple, Metchnikoff suggested that these toxin-producing bacteria could be suppressed by encouraging the growth in the intestine of the lactobacilli from yogurt. His theory was later questioned by bacteriologists who felt that the usual presence of intestinal bile salts might inhibit the proliferation of the "good" bacteria. Nevertheless, many still believe in yogurt's beneficial effects. Additionally, yogurt has recently become popular as a pleasant, low-calorie alternative to ice cream. The introduction of fruit yogurt during the 1940s revolutionized the market. Until recently, yogurt sales increased by 20 percent or so every year.

Commercial yogurt is made by heating concentrated milk, or milk fortified by skim milk powder, to about 90°C (194°F) for a few minutes, then cooling it to about 44°C (111°F), at which point a controlled culture of *Lactobacillus bulgaricus* and *Streptococcus thermophilus* is added. These two lactic organisms produce the required acidity and the delicate yogurt flavor. Souring and thickening take place in about 3 hours at 44°C (111°F), and stop when the mixture is cooled to 5°C (40°F). Because the milk has been heated and soured, and because of its high acidity, pathogens cannot grow in yogurt. It is probably the safest of all perishable foods. Well-made yogurt of any type should last for 14 days if kept at 5°C (41°F).

Many people make their own yogurt. Yogurt makers can be purchased at most large department stores, and they come with complete instructions for home yogurt preparation. They are available in various cup sizes, usually making six one-to-two cup quantities. When you make yogurt yourself, you are the judge of how much sweetener or natural fruits to add and whether to make the yogurt with nonfat or whole milk. Of course, you need the culture to begin your first batch, but after that you can start the next lot from an unused container of the previous batch. We make ours with skim milk and add honey and fresh fruits for sweeteners. It stores well in the refrigerator for several days.

SALADS

Growing your own fruits and vegetables can be really wonderful. The joy of gardening is more than just getting to harvest the best and freshest of table treats. The entire process is nourishing. The steps of gardening include preparing the soil, planting the seeds or seedlings, cultivating and weeding the plot, watering and watching the growth, and finally harvesting the fruits or vegetables. What a joy it is to eat your own home-grown tomato or fruit or to toss a green salad from your fresh picked leaves. Not only does the dish taste better, but there is also no doubt that it is packed with more nutrients. None have been lost during the packaging, storage, shipment, and delivery stages that are unfortunately a part of the contemporary production life. The food goes directly from the harvest to your body. This is the essence of eating living foods. If you have never tried a garden or do not have the space for it, try planting a tomato or two in pots on your patio. You should be pleased with the process and the results.

SUMMARY

Fresh green salads, yogurt, and seed sprouts are examples of living foods. As delicious and healthful as these foods are, there are some cautions involved with their consumption. We need to be aware of potential contamination in some growing and preparation methods. Generally, the more foods are processed, the fewer natural vitamins, minerals, and enzymes remain because cooking, canning, and processing have the capacity to deplete vitamins and mineral stores. In general try to eat food as close as possible to fresh-picked or still living. Remember, living foods offer us an opportunity to ingest vibrant living cells that work to energize our bodies.

REFERENCES

Inami, G. B., Moler, S. E. (1999). Detection and isolation of salmonella from naturally contaminated alfalfa seeds following an outbreak investigation. *Journal of Food Protection, 62*(6), 662–664.

National Advisory Committee on Microbiological Criteria for Foods. (1999). Microbiological safety evaluations and recommendations on sprouted seeds. *International Journal of Food Microbiology, 52*(3), 123–153.

CHAPTER
13

Healing Herbs

Among the various sources of nutrition, there are certain substances that concentrate chemicals and produce particular salutary effects on our body systems. These healing substances are found in herbs. Herbs may be used in small quantities in cooking and food preparation where they add color, flavor, aroma, and zest, as well as in tisanes and teas where they soothe, stimulate, relax, and console us while providing a contemplative and communicative environment. In high concentrations, they may be used therapeutically.

This chapter serves as a brief introduction to the use of herbs. If you would like to pursue this fascinating art, you will probably want to collect individual herb books and begin experimental cultivation of your own small herb garden.

THE SALUTARY EFFECTS OF HERBS

Studying, cultivating, and using herbs can be a transformative process. As you work with herbs, you become more deeply involved with the natural processes and interactions of the healing substances of the earth. You experience the rewards of seeing an organism that you plant and nurture with your own hands transformed by the process of nature. With daily involvement, you become part of birth, dying, rebirth, and transmutation.

Herbalism becomes a holistic process encompassing not only physiological body effects, but those involving the mind, emotions, and spirit. Herbs can be another effective dietary tool when used properly as supplements to food. They aid in the prevention of disease through their ability to modulate and strengthen the immune system.

SOURCES OF HERBS

The best sources of herbs are those that you grow or gather and prepare yourself. This enables you to participate entirely in the process of birth, growth, and transformation of the substance. As you grow or gather herbs, you have the opportunity to experience the true essence of the substance and benefit in multiple ways from the use of it. When herbs are purchased from commercial sources, they should be used in some symbolic way in order to obtain maximum benefit on each level of the body-mind-spirit template.

Growing your own herbs gives you complete control over the environment in which they are grown. You control the soil content, quantity of water, and nutrients, as well as share in the aesthetic process of growth, fruition, and harvest.

When gathering wild herbs, you must know herbs well and harvest far from roads and sources of pollution. Herbs gathered too close to roads will have high concentrations of lead, arsenicals, and other toxins. Some people, such as the Tibetan monks of the high Himalayas, think only wild herbs are useful. Most of us, however, live in a much different environment. Consequently, we must alter our opinions of what is useful.

With the exception of standard teas, when purchasing commercial herbal preparations, it is essential to examine the herb, cross-reference it in an herb book or manual, and use only small quantities until the potency of the preparation can be ascertained.

PREPARING HERBS FOR USE

Several terms are important in understanding the preparation of herbs.

INFUSION

An infusion or a *tisane* is a fancy name for a tea. You can use either fresh (preferable) or dried leaves of the herb (generally three parts fresh is the equivalent of one part dried). Place them into a well-warmed teapot and add about 1 cup of boiling water per 3 teaspoons dried herbs. Then steep the mixture for 10 to 15 minutes. Sweeten the mixture with licorice root, honey, or sugar to make it more palatable. Use infusions immediately; do not store them.

Crushing or grinding the leaves and seeds may enhance the extraction of the volatile oils. You may prefer cold infusions of herbs with highly volatile oils. This is accomplished by placing the herb in a sealed glass container and steeping for a period of 12 hours.

DECOCTION

When the herb used is a hard or woody stem, root, or bark, such as willow, or a hard seed or nut, it is better to use a decoction as opposed to an infusion. The proportions of fresh or dried herbs are the same as with an infusion—3 teaspoons of fresh herb or 1 teaspoon of dried to 1 cup of water. However, after breaking the herb into small pieces, you should simmer it in water in a covered pot for varying periods of time, depending on which herb you are using, and then strain the solution. It is important to use glass vessels rather than metal (especially aluminum) vessels because the boiling of the decoction could extract harmful substances from the metal. The importance of avoiding aluminum cookware in general cannot be overemphasized. The decoction can be refrigerated, but it is best used immediately.

TINCTURES

A tincture is a solution of an herb in an alcohol base. Alcohol is a better solvent and preservative for most plant derivatives than water. Alcohol derivatives of herbs are called tinctures. Preparations can also be made from vinegar and glycerine.

The easiest way to make a tincture is to use vodka or brandy. Place 2 ounces of dried herbs or 4 ounces of fresh herbs in a sealed glass container with 1 cup of vodka or brandy and set the container in a warm place. Shake it periodically. Allow the mixture to steep for 2 to 4 hours and then filter it through a cheesecloth. Tinctures are quite stable and may last for years. You can make tinctures with wine, but they will have a shorter shelf life. For example, rosemary wine can be used as an effective digestive herb.

Tinctures are much stronger than infusions or decoctions. The dosage, therefore, is smaller. Generally, 5 to 15 drops added to hot or cold sweetened water is the best method of using the tincture. Creative herbalists can create their own tarragon, rosemary, or basil vinegars using these herbs in apple cider vinegar.

Syrups for coughs can be made using the appropriate herbs dissolved in a syrup made from a 2-to-3 dilution of sugar and water. The tincture is then added to the sugar syrup in a one-part tincture to three-part syrup mixture.

DRYING HARVESTED HERBS

The most expedient method of drying grown or gathered herbs is to use a commercial dehydrator. The temperature should be set low, about 95°F to 100°F.

A more aesthetic and personal way to dehydrate herbs is by using an ordinary brown paper lunch bag. Prepare the bag by turning down the top to form a cuff. Make several down rolls until the bag is about two-thirds open. Place the herbs in the base of the bag and put it in a warm location, such as on top of the refrigerator. This location allows you to subconsciously notice its presence, which is nice since it reminds you that you are personally involved in the whole process of the preparation. As your herbs dry, the aromas will permeate the surrounding environment. Another method you may want to try is to bundle, tie into a bunch, and hang your herbs from the ceiling or doorway frame. In addition to enjoying the aroma, you will have the aesthetic pleasure of seeing your herbs swaying in the breeze.

Herbs are best stored in airtight, sealed containers. The best containers are corked brown jars. Store the containers in a cool, dark place. For convenience, I store my herbs in ziplock freezer bags in a cool, dark, dry environment.

HERBAL CONSTITUENTS

The substances within herbs are the products and gifts of a fruitful and loving earth. They sustain us by a process of synergism; that is, multiple substances interacting with one another.

Numerous substances, including water, organic and inorganic compounds, sugars, and carbohydrates, are present in herbs. Weak acids are present in herbs such as cranberries. These acids may be useful in the prevention and treatment of urinary tract infections. The "sting" of the nettle plant is related to a weak organic acid.

Some herbs contain alcohol substances. Alcohols such as the menthol in peppermint may be useful in the treatment of respiratory and congestive problems.

Most herbs contain multiple volatile oils that delight our senses, stimulate us, and have therapeutic value. Think of the odors of peppermint, thyme, rosemary, eucalyptus, and garlic. Such oils have both local and systemic effects. After we ingest them, they diffuse to many systems throughout our bodies.

Some of the herbal oils have been found to strengthen our immune systems by a process of "immune modulation." When the herbal substance combines with our internal knowledge systems, it seems to provide our bodies with whatever substance they need, having different effects in different individuals. The effects are modulated not only through our organ systems themselves, but also centrally where the taste and odor of the oil stimulates the olfactory system. This system, which is directly connected with the brain, stimulates feelings of inner peace and well-being, which further modulates the immune mechanism.

Plant sugars and carbohydrates can serve as energy sources and can be used in the process of fermentation. Herbs such as grapes can be made into wines which "gladden" the heart and may produce (in proper quantities) beneficial effects on the cardiac and immune systems.

Phenolic compounds (chemical structures) such as the derivative of willow bark (acetylsalicylic acid or aspirin) and the oil of cloves and thyme are painkillers. The salutary effects of barberry on the urinary tract may be explained by the phenolic compounds. Indeed, a whole new class of antibiotics named the "quinolones" has been based on similar compounds.

Numerous other substances such as tannins, coumanins, glycosides, saponins, and alkaloids are all found in plant substances and interact with one another. Proper and full knowledge of these substances is leading to more incredible medical discoveries each day. For example, digitalis is a cardiac glycoside and coumanins are anticoagulants. When used in small dosages, the effects of these substances can prevent disease and stimulate all our organ systems.

POPULAR HERBS

The following herbs are readily available, either self-grown or obtained at a local health food market.

ALOE

Aloe is easily grown and is best used externally for insect bites, sunburn, and minor burns. It can be used internally as a cathartic, but I do not recommend this.

ANISEED

This can be used as a delicious mystery seasoning in bouillabaisse and seafood dishes. Used medicinally in combination with other herbs, it is effective for treating respiratory problems and is calming to the bowel.

BALM OR LEMON BALM

This can be used in salads, but the most delicious teas are produced from the fresh or dried leaves. I can attest that it has definite calming effects on tensions after a hard day's work. It reduces stress, lightens depression and anxiety, and is effective for digestive disorders. It can be used to supplement lemon verbena and can be combined with most other herbs.

BASIL

Basil can be easily obtained as an annual from most nurseries and adds a delightful touch to salads. My favorite use for it is as a key ingredient in making pesto sauce for fettuccine.

BEARBERRY

Combined with easily gathered yarrow, bearberry can be used as a supplementary treatment for urinary disorders, including gravel (small kidney stones) in the urinary tract.

BORAGE

The use of borage as a tea made from dried leaves is reputed to be a restorative to the adrenal glands and, as such, is said to be effective in chronic stress syndromes. I use the flowers as decorations on salads and the finely chopped leaves directly in the salad. The flavor is somewhat like cucumber with slightly fishy overtones. Consequently, this pungent herb may not be appreciated by everyone. One of its assets is that it is easily grown.

CARAWAY

Caraway is readily available as seeds, which should be crushed to make tea. It is reputed to be effective for flatulence and colic, and when combined with other agents, it may be effective for bronchitis. For zest and texture, add it to your homemade breads. Caraway is the flavorful ingredient in the Scandinavian drink aquavit.

CARDOMOM

These seeds are grown on the Indian subcontinent and provide an interesting effect when used in breads or added to beverages. They can be used medicinally as an appetite stimulant and as a treatment for dyspepsia. This herb is also quite effective when used for respiratory conditions.

CASCARA

Made from treebark, cascara can be used as a mild purgative.

CHAMOMILE

These flowers can be combined in teas to aid in digestion.

CINNAMON

Made from tree bark, cinnamon is a common culinary herb that can also be used to relieve nausea and vomiting and stabilize the bowel.

CLOVES

Cloves are similar in effect to cinnamon. They may also be useful for tooth-aches.

CORIANDER

These seeds are used in pickling spices and, especially when ground, add unique flavor to rice dishes. A coriander rice dish is beneficial to the bowel.

CUCUMBER

Cucumber is delicious in salads, breads, and on fish. The topical application of cucumber juice soothes and cools the skin. Preparations made from cucumber are used in salons for facials.

CUMIN

Similar to coriander, cumin adds warmth to soups and stews, and is an ingredient in curry.

DAMIANA

Tea made with damiana can be used for anxiety and depression. It is said to be a male sexual stimulant.

DANDELION

Dandelion leaves are good in salads. Less commonly used, but equally edible, are the prepared roots. Dandelion can be used medicinally as a powerful diuretic.

DILL

Dill weed and seeds can be used in salads, breads, and on fish. The tea can be used as a remedy for flatulence.

ECHINACEA

This is said to be a good immune system stimulant. The decoction of the root may be helpful in laryngitis and cystitis.

EPHEDRA

Commercially known as MaHuang, ephedra is quite clearly of benefit in asthmatic conditions, as well as allergic problems such as hayfever. This herb must be used with extreme caution, however.

FENNEL

Delicious in salads, fennel is quite flavorful. An infusion of the crushed seeds is helpful in relieving colic and flatulence.

FENUGREEK SEEDS

These seeds are an ancient remedy for localized wounds. The seeds make an interesting tea with a slight hint of curry. The sprouts are exotic when used in salads.

GARLIC

Garlic is the universal "adaptogen" that aids us in many ways. It has antibacterial, antiviral, and antiparasitic properties. It is said to help prevent heart disease and cancer and lower blood pressure and cholesterol levels, and it can be used with other herbs in the treatment of bronchitis and asthma.

GINGER

The roots can be used to produce diaphoresis and to aid digestion.

GENTIAN

Used either as a tincture or a decoction, this root is said to be an appetite stimulant.

GINSENG

The roots have been firmly established in the medical literature as an adaptogen. The regular use of ginseng as an infusion or decoction is said to be an antidepressant and improves physical and mental performance.

HAWTHORNE

When used in the proper mixture and proportions, these berries have been found to reduce blood pressure.

HOPS

The hops flowers are an excellent treatment for insomnia, especially when combined with valerian. The shelf life for the flowers is quite limited.

HORSERADISH

Horseradish makes an excellent sauce when ground. It can be used as an infusion that is helpful in influenza and fevers as well as in bronchitis.

HORSETAIL

This is commonly available along paths and roads. The dried stems and leaves can be made into an infusion that is helpful in the treatment of prostate problems. When combined with saw palmetto berries, it may actually be able to shrink enlarged prostates. However, the scientific information about this use is scant.

JUNIPER

The berries add an interesting flavor to wild game and to rice and wheat pilafs. The infusion is said to be helpful in rheumatism and cystitis, but should be avoided in kidney disease. Medically, it should be used with caution.

LAVENDER

Lavender is delightful to the eye and has a lovely aroma. The flowers and leaves are used in potpourris. The oil can be rubbed on the skin, but avoid any internal use, even in salads.

LICORICE

Made from the glycerrhiza root (meaning sweet root), licorice can be used as the basis of many infusions and delightful teas. When combined with other herbs, it is effective as a treatment for bronchitis. It also has salutary effects on the gastrointestinal system. Its overuse, however, should be avoided by persons with high blood pressure.

MARJORAM

Easily grown, marjoram makes an excellent addition to stews, salads, and soups. Infusions from marjoram may be useful for headaches.

MULLEIN

The flower is steeped in hot water until the water is yellow. The tea relieves persistent cough, respiratory mucus, and hoarseness.

MUSTARD

The seeds, when crushed in warm water, are used to induce vomiting. Mustard is used in powdered form to make a poultice that draws blood to the skin and relieves pain and inflammation in rheumatism and arthritis.

These are but a few of the healing herbs. Many others such as nasturtium, nettles, oats, parsley, peppermint, pumpkin, raspberry, red clover, red sage, rose hips, rosemary, saw palmetto, thyme, valerian, and yarrow all have healing medicinal uses.

CAUTIONS ABOUT USING HERBS

Herbal remedies are becoming increasingly popular among patients as treatment for such varied medical problems as arthritis, depression, diabetes, menstrual irregularity, and pulmonary conditions. However, herbal preparations can have many negative effects so they must be used with caution. With the current lack of standardization and control there will likely be contamination and toxicity of herbal products and potential side effects associated with various herbs (Borins, 1998). For example, Chinese-herb nephropathy is a progressive form of renal fibrosis that develops in some patients who take weight-reducing pills containing Chinese herbs. Because of a manufacturing error, one of the herbs in these pills *(Stephania tetrandra)* was inadvertently replaced by *Aristolochia fangchi,* which is nephrotoxic and carcinogenic (Nortier et al., 2000). This cruel, terminal illness shows what can happen without rigorous checks and controls in the herbal manufacturing business. There are so many possible negative side effects from the misuse of herbs coming to light that even the popular press is warning consumers to beware (Fischman, 2000). Even the most common herbs, kava, St. John's wort, and ginkgo have untoward effects when used inappropriately (Waddell, Hummel, & Sumners, 2001).

Other cautions include self-dosage and preparation. For example, when formulating your own teas and compounds, refer to at least three different reference sources to validate the safety of your recipe. Some common herbs, such as angelica and sassafras, can be carcinogenic. Other commonly used herbs, such as saffron, can be toxic to the heart and liver in high concentrations. Foxglove, from which digitalis was originally made, can in very minute dosages stimulate the heart, but in slightly higher doses, it can produce cardiac arrhythmias and has been incriminated in numerous fatalities. On the other hand, with the proper knowledge, herbs can serve both as supplements for healing and in the prevention of illness and disease.

SUMMARY

Growing, harvesting, eating, consuming, and discussing herbs has been very popular during the past decade. Everywhere you look there are books and articles on this provocative and innovative topic. Studying, cultivating, and using herbs can contribute to personal empowerment. In your enthusiasm for using herbs, do be aware of the increasing number of cautions and precautions, and use wise professional judgment before recommending them to clients or friends or using them yourself.

Herbalism can be a holistic process engaging all our physical senses while at the same time involving our minds and spirits. Herbs used in the proper doses and mixtures can be among the most healing of all our foods.

REFERENCES

Borins, M. (1998). The dangers of using herbs. What your patients need to know. *Postgraduate Medicine, 104*(1), 91–95, 99–100.

Fischman, J. (2000). Herbs and prescriptions can make a risky mixture. *U.S. News and World Report, 128*(17), 64–65.

Nortier, J. L., Martinez, M. C., Schmeiser, H. H., Arlt, V. M., Bieler, C. A., Petein, M., Depierreux, M. F., De Pauw, L., Abramowicz, D., Vereerstraeten, P., & Vanherweghem, J. L. (2000). Urothelial carcinoma associated with the use of a Chinese herb. *New England Journal of Medicine, 342*(23), 1686–1692.

Waddell, D. L., Hummel, M. E., & Sumners, A. D. (2001). Three herbs you should get to know. *American Journal of Nursing, 101*(4), 48–54.

CHAPTER 14

Vegetarianism

People who abstain from foods of animal origin are vegetarians. The first of several subcategories include those who refer to themselves as vegans and avoid all animal foods. The second group, the lacto-ovo-vegetarians, allow eggs and dairy products in their diets. Because egg whites and some dairy products are outstanding protein sources and fair sources of vitamin B_{12}, the lacto-ovo-vegetarian diet can easily be a nutritious one. A true vegan diet, without eggs and dairy products, takes greater attention, planning, and knowledge to maintain adequate nutritional intake and optimal health. Unbalanced vegetarian diets can result in scurvy, anemia, protein starvation, and death. A third variation of the vegetarian diet is the macrobiotic diet, which includes whole grains, legumes, vegetables, and other staples of the Eastern world. Technically, macrobiotic followers may not be true vegetarians if they include some fish and seafood products in their diet.

A new area of interest is *vegetarian awareness*. This term indicates a necessary understanding by those of us who deal with foods. We all probably know people who are vegetarians. If we do not understand this dietary variation, we probably wonder about the adequacy of their diet, the reasons for their variation, and why and how they eat in this way.

HISTORY

Although this mode of nutrition has had a limited historical practice in North America, it has been followed for centuries in places such as the Asian subcontinent. However, vegetarianism is not historically restricted to the East. The sixth-century

Greek philosopher Pythagoras and others abstained from meat eating based primarily on their beliefs in the transmigration of souls. In the 18th century, Benjamin Franklin in America and Voltaire in France were prominent advocates of vegetarianism. Although there have always been followers of this practice, the rapid growth of this movement in the United States has occurred chiefly since the 1970s. Today there are millions of practicing vegetarians, with books, journals, seminars, and meetings to aid them in the pursuit of clean, wholesome, healthful eating.

Social Aspects of Vegetarianism

A group of researchers looked for the symbolic meaning of eating by comparing the values and beliefs of vegetarians and omnivores. They compared a wide range of vegetarians and omnivores on right-wing authoritarianism, social dominance orientation, human values, and consumption values. The participants tending toward omnivorism differed from those leaning toward veganism and vegetarianism in two principal ways: The omnivores (1) were more likely to endorse hierarchical domination and (2) placed less importance on emotional states. Accordingly, the acceptance or rejection of meat covaried with the acceptance or rejection of the values associated with meat; that finding suggests that individuals consume meat and embrace its symbolism in ways consistent with their self-definitions (Allen, Wilson, Ng, & Dunne, 2000).

WHY BE A VEGETARIAN?

There are several reasons why people subscribe to vegetarianism. Perhaps the primary one is related to religious beliefs. In religions that affirm a belief in reincarnation, a multilife kinship between humans and animals, the eating of flesh is forbidden. The belief is that if you do not surmount certain problems in this life, then it is possible to be born again in the lower life-form of an animal. Since you would not want to take the chance of consuming a friend or relative, or having your heirs consume you, then eating any animal flesh is taboo.

A second reason people adhere to a diet devoid of meat relates to their environmental concerns. People concerned about the ability of the planet to produce sufficient quantities of food to sustain a burgeoning population think that reducing meat consumption will help. For example, an acre of land will yield a much greater quantity of edible plant food than animal meat. An acre of land can produce as much as 385 pounds of alfalfa seed from 1 pound of seed. If 384 pounds were sprouted for food, the yield would be approximately 3,180 pounds of consumable sprouts. Thus, we can see why consumption of protein-containing sprouted food could make a significant environmental difference.

A third reason for vegetarianism relates to health. Many advocates of this lifestyle are queasy about the sanitation of production houses, slaughter methods, and possible contamination of the meat itself during the transportation, storage, and preparation process.

In the United States, approximately 1 million farmers and ranchers raise livestock, which are slaughtered at approximately 6,000 federally inspected plants, that do more than 97 percent of all processing. Currently, four major packers process approximately 70 percent of the beef and another four about 60 percent of the pork in the United States. Although the Humane Slaughter Act (1960) requires that prior to slaughter animals be rendered completely unconscious with a minimum of excitement and discomfort using mechanical, electrical, or chemical (carbon dioxide gas) methods, some people contend that this practice is not followed as closely as it should be.

The Seventh-Day Adventist religious community comprises an enormous group of vegetarians worldwide. To support their tenets on the health benefits of this lifestyle, they continually collect data to demonstrate its benefits. They contend that

- Adventist men 55 and over who eat meat 6 or more times a week are twice as likely to die of heart disease as vegetarian Adventists.
- Adventist men age 40 to 54 who eat meat 6 or more times a week have 4 times the risk of a fatal heart attack than do vegetarian Adventists.
- Adventist meat-eating women over 55 have 1.5 times the risk of a fatal heart attack than do female vegetarian Adventists.

Even the conservative American Dietetic Association recognizes that a growing body of scientific evidence supports a positive relationship between the consumption of a plant-based diet and the prevention of certain diseases. The meat industry denies the health benefits of vegetarian diets, but research on cancer, heart disease, high blood pressure, diabetes, and obesity might lead us to argue otherwise. The average blood cholesterol level of vegetarians is about 125, which is much lower than that of average Americans. Because they eat less fat and more grains, legumes, and vegetables, vegetarians appear to be healthier than average Americans.

ADEQUACY OF NUTRIENTS IN THE DIET

It is quite possible for vegetarians to obtain all the nutrients they need. Studies conducted at the University of Belgium at the beginning of the 20th century compared endurance, strength, and quickness of recovery from fatigue in vegetarians and meat eaters. The findings indicated that vegetarians were superior in all three characteristics. Replicated studies in 1907 at Yale University and in 1909 at Battle Creek Sanitarium in Michigan confirmed the original findings.

Lacto-ovo-vegetarians gained international recognition in 1917–1918 during World War I when a group of captive Danes were deprived of meat and forced to subsist on grains, fruits, and dairy products. To the great surprise of their captors, they exhibited improved health and lowered death rates.

Amino Acids

In the early 1900s chemical analysis of foods began to provide a scientific basis for nutrition. The essential amino acids were determined, vitamins were isolated, and minerals were identified. Protein is an essential element in the diet. The amino acid building blocks must be available to the cytoplasm. Many amino acids are synthesized in our bodies, but some are not. Those not synthesized are called essential. They include isoleucine, leucine, lysine, methionine, phenylalanine, threonine, tryptophan, and valine. These amino acids must be obtained from the foods we eat.

One of the potential problems in vegetarianism is that nearly all types of vegetable protein are deficient in certain essential amino acids. The notable exception is soybeans. That is why this food is one of the essential ingredients in the vegan's diet. In addition to using soybeans, certain foods can be combined throughout the day to create complete proteins. For example, eating corn and beans, rice and beans, or coupling certain cereals with legumes produces a complete protein.

Knowing this information helps health professionals to teach good vegetarian eating combinations. In the southern United States and Mexico, for example, corn is a staple. If people ate corn alone, their diets would be deficient in tryptophan and lysine, and their growth and tissue replacement would be impaired. By combining corn with beans, vegans can balance their diets. Vegetarian peoples of interior Africa and India tend to suffer from protein deficiencies that their coastal brothers and sisters avoid because coastal residents supplement their diets with fish. In these areas, there is a significant need for nutritional teaching utilizing locally available foods.

One possible hazard of the vegan diet is an extreme reduction in saturated fat and cholesterol intake. Our bodies do produce their own cholesterol when it is not ingested; but we require a certain level of fat intake to maintain homeostasis and for the absorption of fat-soluble vitamins. The upside of this issue is that vegetarians may have a lower risk for coronary artery disease since they do not have the saturated fat intake to build up atherosclerotic plaques along their vessel walls.

ADVANTAGES AND DISADVANTAGES OF VEGETARIAN DIETS

Advantages

While there may be some disadvantages to a vegetarian diet, there are specific advantages. These include:

- Increased fiber. Vegetables and fruits are high in fiber compared to fleshy meat. Increased fiber aids in bowel movements and helps to prevent problems such as diverticulitis and colon cancer.
- Decreased daily caloric intake. Vegetables tend to be low in calories, so a vegetarian diet is beneficial to people trying to maintain or lose weight.
- Decreased total fat, saturated fat, and cholesterol intake. Because fruits and vegetables are low in fat and cholesterol compared to meat, vegetarian diets can be beneficial to people with hyperlipidemia (elevated level of lipids in the blood) and can decrease the risk of developing atherosclerosis.
- Financial economy. Meat is often expensive. A vegetarian diet provides an affordable source of protein.

Possible Disadvantages

- Protein deficiency. See pages 175–176 in this chapter on combining grains and legumes.
- Flatulence. When you begin a vegetarian diet, the bowel needs time to adjust to the increased amount of fiber. Until the bowel adjusts to a slower rate, frequent bowel movements and flatus may occur. However, new products are available that can be added in small amounts to food servings. These derivatives of molds can aid in digestion, thus decreasing flatulence. If you are allergic to medicines such as penicillin, however, you should probably avoid these products because you might be allergic to the antigas formula as well. One commercially available product for this condition is Beano™.

CURRENT RESEARCH ON VEGETARIANISM

Health Aspects

The Seventh-Day Adventists comprise a major group of vegetarians in the United States. Epidemiologic studies have shown that their dietary habits are associated with lower risk of coronary heart disease (CHD) and other chronic diseases. However, there are some other interesting findings. Meat consumption is clearly hazardous for Adventist men by raising CHD mortality; however, it is curious that no such effect is seen in women. Data strongly support the role of nuts as protective for CHD. It may be that consumption of modest quantities of certain fats is beneficial rather than hazardous. The lower risk of CHD in Adventists probably has a complicated explanation and certainly cannot be entirely explained by their nonsmoking status or a superior serum lipid profile (Fraser, 1999).

Vegetarian Women

One study compared the risk of ischemic heart disease among older vegetarian Chinese women with that of older nonvegetarian women. Ninety vegetarian Chinese women older than 70 in Hong Kong were screened for ischemic heart disease by electrocardiogram (ECG) and cardiovascular questionnaire. They were compared with 90 nonvegetarian women of similar age examined in a previous local survey. The percentage of subjects with ischemic heart disease defined by symptoms and ECG or by ECG alone was significantly lower among vegetarian women. Vegetarians had lower serum cholesterol levels: more were old age home residents and were less likely to perform regular exercise. Apart from lower serum cholesterol levels, vegetarianism may have other protective factors against ischemic heart disease (Kwok, Woo, Ho, & Sham, 2000).

Few controlled trials have studied cholesterol-lowering diets in premenopausal women. None has examined the cholesterol-lowering effect of a low-fat vegetarian diet, which, in other population groups, leads to marked reductions in serum cholesterol concentrations and, in combination with other lifestyle changes, a regression of atherosclerosis. Researchers tested the hypothesis that a low-fat, vegetarian diet significantly reduces serum total and low-density lipoprotein (LDL) cholesterol concentrations in premenopausal women. In a crossover design, 35 women, age 22 to 48, followed a low-fat vegetarian diet deriving approximately 10 percent of energy from fat for two menstrual cycles. For two additional cycles, they followed their customary diet while also taking a supplement, which was actually a placebo. Serum lipid concentrations were assessed at baseline and during each intervention phase. The findings were that in healthy premenopausal women, a low-fat vegetarian diet led to rapid and sizable reductions in serum total, LDL, and HDL cholesterol concentrations (Barnard et al., 2000).

Adolescents and Young Adults

Young adults frequently experiment with vegetarian and weight-loss diets. Comparisons of their experiences on different diets may help in the development of approaches to improve long-term adherence to weight-loss regimens. In a recent study vegetarian and weight-loss diets were compared on how long and how strictly they were followed, and the reasons why they were initiated and discontinued. From 428 college students surveyed, four groups were delineated:

1. participants who followed a vegetarian diet but not a weight-loss diet (59 Vegetarians),

2. participants who tried a weight-loss diet but not a vegetarian diet (117 Weight-Loss subjects),

3. participants who followed both a vegetarian and a weight-loss diet (133 Both), and

4. participants who had not tried either diet (119 Neither).

The differences were examined by comparing the Vegetarian and Weight-Loss groups as well as by comparing the two diets within the Both group. Duration of the vegetarian diet was much greater than the weight-loss diet; most participants in the Vegetarian group (62 percent) remained on their diet for more than 1 year, whereas the majority of the Weight-Loss participants (61 percent) followed their diet for 1 to 3 months. Similar results were found when comparing the two diets within the Both group. How strictly the two diets were followed, however, did not differ. Analyses revealed that reasons for discontinuing a diet varied; participants were more likely to cite boredom as a reason for discontinuing a weight-loss diet than a vegetarian diet. The longer duration of the vegetarian diet relative to the weight-loss diet warrants further investigation. Results could possibly be applied to behavioral weight-loss treatment to improve long-term maintenance (Smith, Burke, & Wing, 2000).

A cobalamin (Vitamin B_{12}) deficiency has been described in children consuming macrobiotic diets. Some deficiencies include a sore tongue, weakness, fatigue, weight loss, back pain, and apathy. Researchers investigated whether moderate consumption of animal products is sufficient for achieving normal cobalamin function in 73 adolescents who had received a macrobiotic diet until 6 years of age and had then switched to a lacto-vegetarian, lacto-ovo-vegetarian, or omnivorous diet. Data from 94 age-matched adolescents who received an omnivorous diet from birth were used as a reference. Findings were that serum cobalamin concentrations were significantly lower. In macrobiotic adolescents, dairy products (200 g milk or yogurt and 22 g cheese per day) supplied on average 0.95 microg cobalamin per day; additionally, these adolescents consumed fish, meat, or chicken 2 to 3 times a week. In girls, meat consumption contributed more to cobalamin status than the consumption of dairy products, whereas in boys these food groups were equally important. A substantial number of the formerly strict macrobiotic adolescents still had impaired cobalamin function. Thus, moderate consumption of animal products is not sufficient for restoring normal cobalamin status in subjects with inadequate cobalamin intake during the early years of life (van Dusseldorp et al., 1999).

Zinc Intake and Vegetarians

Every day, vegetarians consume many carbohydrate-rich plant foods such as fruits and vegetables, cereals, legumes, and nuts. As a consequence, their diet contains more antioxidant vitamins (vitamin C, vitamin E, and beta-carotene) and copper than that of omnivores. Intake of zinc is generally comparable to that of omnivores. However, the bioavailability of zinc in vegetarian diets is generally lower than that of omnivores. Dietary intake of selenium is variable in both groups and depends on the selenium content of the soil in which the vegetables are grown. Measurements of antioxidant body levels in vegetarians show that a vegetarian diet maintains higher antioxidant vitamin status (vitamin C, vitamin E, beta-carotene) but variable antioxidant trace element status as compared with an omnivorous diet (Rauma & Mykkanen, 2000).

Vegetarians have a lower incidence of many chronic diseases than omnivores. However, vegetarian diets can result in lower intakes of some minerals, particularly zinc. In one cross-sectional study, dietary zinc intake was measured using 12-day weighed records from 99 vegetarians (10 vegans) age 18 to 50 years and 49 age- and sex-matched omnivores. In men, the mean daily zinc intake and zinc density values were similar in omnivores, lacto-ovo-vegetarians, and vegans, but in women they were significantly lower in vegetarians and few achieved the recommended intake. Significantly more vegetarian than omnivorous women had a daily zinc intake of less than 6 mg. Mean serum zinc concentrations were similar in female omnivores and vegetarians, despite the differences in intake. However, omnivorous men had a lower mean serum zinc concentration and more subjects had levels below the reference range than lacto-ovo-vegetarians. Overall, more women than men had low zinc concentrations; and these women generally had intakes below 6 mg a day. There was a significant correlation between serum zinc concentration and dietary zinc density in vegetarians, especially females, but not in omnivores. Lacto-ovo-vegetarians did not have a significantly greater risk of low zinc status than omnivores (Ball & Ackland, 2000).

Vegan Proteins Promote Increased Glucagon Activity

Amino acids modulate the secretion of both insulin and glucagon; the composition of dietary protein therefore has the potential to influence the balance of glucagon and insulin activity. Soy protein, as well as many other vegan proteins, are higher in nonessential amino acids than most animal-derived food proteins, and as a result should preferentially favor glucagon production. Acting on hepatocytes, glucagon promotes (and insulin inhibits) cAMP-dependent mechanisms that down-regulate lipogenic enzymes and cholesterol synthesis, while up-regulating hepatic LDL receptors and production of the IGF-I antagonist IGFBP-1. The insulin-sensitizing properties of many vegan diets—high in fiber, low in saturated fat—should amplify these effects by down-regulating insulin secretion. Additionally, the relatively low essential amino acid content of some vegan diets may decrease hepatic IGF-I synthesis. Thus, diets featuring vegan proteins can be expected to lower elevated serum lipid levels, promote weight loss, and decrease circulating IGF-I activity. The latter effect should impede cancer induction (as is seen in animal studies with soy protein), lessen neutrophil-mediated inflammatory damage, and slow growth and maturation in children.

In fact, vegans tend to have low serum lipids, lean physiques, shorter stature, later puberty, and decreased risk for certain prominent Western cancers; a vegan diet has documented clinical efficacy in rheumatoid arthritis. Low-fat vegan diets may be especially protective in regard to cancers linked to insulin resistance—namely, breast and colon cancer—as well as prostate cancer; conversely, the high IGF-I activity associated with heavy ingestion of animal products may be largely responsible for the epidemic of Western cancers in wealthy societies. Increased phytochemical intake is also likely to contribute to the reduction of cancer risk in vegans. Regression of coronary stenoses has been documented during low-fat vegan diets coupled with exercise training; such regimens also tend to markedly improve diabetic control and lower elevated blood pressure. Risk of many other degenerative disorders may be decreased in vegans, although reduced growth factor activity may be responsible for an increased risk of hemorrhagic stroke. By altering the glucagon/insulin balance, it is conceivable that supplemental intakes of key nonessential amino acids could enable omnivores to enjoy some of the health advantages of a vegan diet. An unnecessarily high intake of essential amino acids, either in the absolute sense or relative to total dietary protein, may prove to be as grave a risk factor for Western degenerative diseases as is excessive fat intake (McCarty, 1999).

Vegan Diet–Based Lifestyle Program Lowers Homocysteine Levels

Plasma homocysteine levels have been directly associated with cardiac disease risk. Current research raises concerns as to whether comprehensive lifestyle approaches including a plant-based diet may interact with other known modulators of homocysteine levels. Researchers reported observations of homocysteine levels in 40 self-selected subjects who participated in a vegan diet–based lifestyle program. Each subject attended a residential lifestyle change program and had fasting plasma total homocysteine measured on enrollment and then after 1 week of lifestyle intervention. The intervention included a vegan diet, moderate physical exercise, stress management and spirituality enhancement sessions, group support, and exclusion of tobacco, alcohol, and caffeine. B vitamin supplements known to reduce blood homocysteine levels were not provided. Subjects' mean homocysteine levels fell 13 percent. Subgroup analysis showed that homocysteine decreased across a range of demographic and diagnostic categories. These results suggest that broad-based lifestyle interventions favorably impact homocysteine levels (DeRose et al., 2000).

WHAT TO EAT

Most new vegans quickly learn the proper balance of whole grains, vegetables, fruits, legumes, nuts, and seeds. These people generally do not waste any part of their daily caloric intake on empty calories such as candy, cakes, sodas, or other foods that have no nutritional value.

The Macrobiotic Diet

Macrobiotics refers to a way of eating based on choosing and preparing foods in harmony with nature and in accordance with our individual needs. By promoting a diet low in fat, high in complex carbohydrates and fiber, and nearly cholesterol-free, macrobiotics support the concept of the link between healthy diet and healthy lifestyle.

In the macrobiotic diet, all foods are categorized as either yin (expansive, relaxing, or diffusive) or yang (contractive or having a focused effect). Meat and salt, for example, are highly contractive yang foods. In a meal containing these foods, more expansive yin foods such as vegetables should be eaten to bring the contractive foods into balance. Advocates of this regimen believe that an excessive yang diet can result in overly contractive physical or emotional tendencies, such as hypertension or feeling uptight. At the opposite extreme, an overly yin diet can make us feel unmotivated or uncoordinated physically and emotionally. The goal in macrobiotics is to avoid either extreme and to eat foods that are more balanced within themselves and to one another. Within this system, food should also be balanced with activity level and the weather. For example, on a cold day, you drink warm teas to balance the temperature. Even illnesses are categorized as yin or yang and are balanced accordingly with proper food and treatment.

Those who follow a macrobiotic diet seek food in its most natural state: fresh, locally grown, when possible, without chemical fertilizers or pesticides, and free of additives and preservatives. Dairy products and highly refined carbohydrates are discouraged.

The standard macrobiotic diet usually consists of 50 percent grains, 25 percent vegetables, 5 to 10 percent beans and sea vegetables, 5 percent soup, and 5 percent condiments and other foods. Whole grains, including brown rice, millet, barley, oats, buckwheat, quinoa, rye, amaranth, corn, and whole wheat are cooked with sea salt to enhance digestibility. For optimum nutrition, whole grains are preferable to white breads and noodles.

Depending on the climate, season, and our individual needs, it is suggested that at least two-thirds of the vegetables be steamed, boiled, baked, or sautéed, while one-third may be eaten raw. Persons living in temperate zones should consume vegetables and fruits grown in a similar climate or, preferably, the same region. Nonindigenous foods such as bananas, pineapple, and even potatoes and tomatoes are not recommended for frequent use.

Sea vegetables are especially high in minerals such as calcium. They can be cooked with beans, soups, and vegetables or made into side dishes cooked and seasoned with soy sauce.

Soup made with fermented soybean paste called miso (pronounced "mee-so") is generally eaten on a daily basis. Unpasteurized miso is abundant in lactobacillus bacteria and enzymes, which reportedly aid digestion and food assimilation. Miso should be added to soup stock at the end of cooking and should not be boiled. This preserves the "good" bacteria and the enzymes.

Condiments, especially sesame salt (commonly known as gomasio; pronounced "go-mah-see-o"), are used to enhance flavor, add nutrition, promote better digestion, and help balance the meal with regard to the yin and yang. Traditional pickles such as daikon radish, sauerkraut, and rice bran are an important part of this whole grain-based diet.

Twig tea, barley tea, grain coffees, and noncarbonated mineral water are the beverages of choice in the macrobiotic diet.

Soybeans

Soybeans are one of the most important sources of protein known to humankind. Soybean crops can produce over 33 percent more protein from an acre of land than any other known crop and 20 times as much usable protein as can be raised on an acre of land used for grazing cattle. The yield of protein is high, both in terms of quantity and quality. Soybeans contain about 35 percent protein, more than any other unprocessed plant or animal food. Another exceptional quality of soy protein is that it includes all of the eight essential amino acids in a configuration readily usable by the human body. For example, a ½-cup serving of usable soy protein is equivalent to 5 ounces of steak. The difference between the two is that the soybeans have no cholesterol or saturated fats.

Soy protein–containing foods are a rich source of isoflavone phytoestrogens, such as genistein and daidzein. There is great interest in these substances because lower rates of chronic diseases, including coronary heart disease, have been associated with high dietary intake of soy-containing foods. Soy phytoestrogens bind weakly to estrogen receptors, and some bind more strongly to estrogen receptor-beta compared with estrogen receptor-alpha. A meta-analysis has indicated that isoflavone phytoestrogens lowered plasma cholesterol concentrations in subjects with initially elevated levels, but had little effect in subjects with normal cholesterol concentrations (Tikkanen & Adlercreutz, 2000).

There are two issues related to soybeans that are important to consider:

1. Some thyroid specialist contend that some people have an adverse response to high soybean intake. These are people challenged by autoimmune low thyroid condition, which includes 12 percent of the general population and 20 percent of menopausal women. The adverse response is lowered thyroid function due to genistein (one of the isoflavones found in soy) blocking the action of iodine and tyrosine in the production of thyroid

hormone. Also, in adults, soy products appear to elevate T-4 without modifying T-3, thereby upsetting the important T-3/T-4 ratio. This can result in weight gain as well as low thyroid function (Osborn, 1999; Shames & Shames, 2001; Wood et al., 1995).

2. Approximately 60 percent of the soybeans sold in the United States have been genetically modified (GM). Currently there is no requirement in the United States, as there is in European countries, to label GM foods. To date there is no scientific data on the effect of long-term use of GM foods on the human body.

The United States now produces about two-thirds of the world's soybeans. Actually, soybeans are one of our largest crops, second only to corn and wheat. Enough soybeans are grown each year to provide every American with their full RDA/DRI requirements for three years. If the soybeans produced in the United States were distributed equally among all the people on the planet, they would fulfill about 25 percent of their yearly protein requirements. However, the vast majority of these soybeans never reach human beings. They are exported, extracted for oil, or used as feed for livestock.

Almost all of America's nonexported soybeans go to factories where millions of pounds a day are converted to soy oil. This oil, which contains no protein, is refined and sold as cooking or salad oil. Defatted soybean meal is the primary by-product of the oil extraction process. This meal contains about 2½ times as much protein by weight as steak. What happens to the meal? It is fed to livestock. In addition to this prize protein, we feed livestock 78 percent of all our grain. Both the soybeans and the grain could be used directly as food for people. As a society, we have yet to understand and utilize soybeans as an important food source.

The soybeans utilized for human consumption are hallmarks of many vegetarian diets. The foods derived from soybeans are tofu, miso (fermented soybean paste), and shoyu (natural soy sauce). Miso is often served as a soup and shoyu is used as a high-protein seasoning. Tofu is used as the backbone of the vegetarian diet in much the same way as meat and dairy products are used in the typical American diet.

Tofu is a colorless bean curd that comes in a variety of shapes and forms and can be cut, fried, baked, or ground to use in any cooking combination. It is prepared by a process that removes the crude fiber, making it much easier to digest than the meats and grains we ordinarily eat. Babies, the elderly, and people with digestive problems can thrive on tofu.

Tofu is low in calories. An 8-ounce serving of eggs has about 450 calories. An 8-ounce serving of meat has about 600 calories, while the same amount of tofu contains only 150 calories. We know there is a correlation between overweight and consumption of large amounts of animal foods high in saturated fats. Research studies show that American vegetarians are 20 pounds below the national average. In countries with relatively low meat consumption, such as Japan and India, people are close to the ideal body weights.

We know that herbicides, pesticides, and heavy metals tend to concentrate in the fatty tissues of animals at the top of the food chain. Fish, poultry, and meat contain about 20 times more pesticide residues than legumes. Because soybeans are a legume crop at the base of the food chain, their spraying is carefully monitored by the Food and Drug Administration to keep the level of contamination at a minimum. Soybean foods in the diet have been found to lower the risk of breast cancer in premenopausal women (Cassidy, Bingham, & Setchell, 1995). In general, soy products have been found to be helpful in preventing colon, prostate, and breast cancer (Messina & Barnes, 1991).

There are many reasons to use tofu in our diets. Tofu is

- an excellent source of calcium—an 8-ounce serving provides 38 percent RDA of calcium.
- an excellent source of iron, phosphorus, potassium, sodium, essential B vitamins, choline, and fat-soluble vitamin E.
- a high-quality protein.
- easy to digest.
- low in saturated fats and cholesterol.
- free of chemical toxins.
- helpful for preventing cancer.
- low in cost.
- versatile and easy to use.

Buying and Using Tofu

Most grocery stores now carry tofu. It is often found in the fresh produce section or in the refrigerator section near the dairy products. Fresh packaged tofu comes in a plastic container with a date stamped on the outside. Buy tofu with the most recent date; if an expiration date has been reached, do not buy it. Ask the produce manager to get fresh tofu from the storeroom. If none is available, postpone your purchase.

After you bring your fresh tofu home from the store, keep it under constant refrigeration until you are ready to use it. If you must postpone preparing your dish for several days, you can store tofu by slitting the top of the plastic seal, draining the water contents, and refilling the package around the tofu with new water. You can drain and refill for up to 10 days without product spoilage. There will be some loss of texture and flavor, but the nutrient value will remain intact.

TABLE 14–1	**Tofu Meal Ideas**

Breakfast
Butter-fried tofu
Scrambled tofu eggs
Pan-fried tofu
Tofu fruit whips

Desserts
Fresh fruit salad with tofu whipped cream
Tofu peanut butter and banana spread
Tofu cheesecake
Tofu pudding

Lunch and Dinner Dishes
Tofu spaghetti sauce
Tofu cottage cheese
Carrot and raisin salad with tofu
Tofu guacamole
Tofu burgers
Curried rice with tofu
Crisp deep-fried tofu
Chunky tofu and pineapple

Once you begin cooking with tofu, you will awaken to a world of recipes and uses for this versatile food. You will discover dishes that can be enjoyed from breakfast to dinners to desserts. With tofu, you can create sauces, soups, toppings, dressings, stocks, and entrées. Table 14–1 gives you a few ideas.

CURRENT SOYBEAN RESEARCH

Soybean Diet and Coronary Heart Disease

Epidemiological studies, and some clinical trials, demonstrate that a proper diet reduces the rate of occurrence of cardiovascular disorders. Several in vitro studies suggest that some components of plant foods, most of which share a phenolic structure, are endowed with interesting pharmacological activities. There is evidence that correlates high dietary intake of phytochemicals from various sources with a reduced incidence of coronary heart disease (Visioli, Borsani, & Galli, 2000).

Soybean Consumption and Breast Cancer

Ovarian hormones are biomarkers for breast cancer risk. Soybean consumption may be responsible in part for lower levels of ovarian hormones and decreased rates of breast cancer in women in Asia compared with Western populations. Soybeans contain a significant amount of the isoflavones daidzein and genistein, which are weak estrogens. One study was undertaken to determine whether soya feeding decreases circulating levels of ovarian hormones and gonadotropins. Ten healthy, regularly cycling women consumed a constant soya-containing diet on a metabolic unit, starting on day 2 of a menstrual cycle until day 2 of the next cycle. Blood and urine samples were obtained daily for one menstrual cycle before and during soy feeding. The diet was calculated to maintain constant body weight, included 400 kilocalories from a 36-ounce portion of soymilk, and provided 113 to 207 mg a day of total isoflavones. For the group, the soya diet provided more carbohydrate and less protein than the home diets. Daily consumption of the soya diet reduced circulating levels of 17beta-estradiol by 25 percent and of progesterone by 45 percent compared with levels during the home diet period but had no effect on luteinizing hormone or follicle-stimulating hormone. Mean menstrual cycle length did not change during the soya diet. Consumption of an isoflavone-containing soya diet reduced levels of ovarian steroids in normal women over the entire menstrual cycle without affecting gonadotropins. This suggests that at least under the conditions of this study, soya-induced reductions of circulating ovarian steroids are not mediated by gonadotropins. Decreases in ovarian hormones are related to isoflavones contained in soy and also to energy intake and other components such as protein and fiber but not fat. These results may explain decreased ovarian hormone levels and decreased risk of breast cancer in populations consuming soya diets and have implications for reducing breast cancer risk by dietary intervention (Lu, Anderson, Grady, Kohen, & Nagamani, 2000).

Breast cancer is the most common cancer in women. Because genetics is believed to account for only 10 to 15 percent of breast cancer cases, the environment, including nutrition, is thought to play a significant role in predisposing women to this disease. Studies of Asian women suggest that those who consume a traditional diet high in soy products have a low incidence of breast cancer, but that among emigrants to the United States, the second generation, but not the first, loses this protection. These findings suggest a possible common mechanism of action for breast cancer protection from early, specific nutritional exposure. Genistein, an isoflavone found in soy, has been reported to have weak estrogenic and antiestrogenic properties, to be an antioxidant, to inhibit topoisomerase II and angiogenesis, and to induce cell differentiation. Researchers hypothesize that the early genistein action promotes cell differentiation that results in a less active epidermal growth factor signaling pathway in adulthood that, in turn, suppresses the development of mammary cancer. These researchers speculate that breast cancer protection in Asian women consuming a traditional soy-containing diet is derived from early exposure to soybean products containing genistein, and believe that early events are essential for the benefits of cancer protection (Lamartiniere, 2000).

Soy Diet Effects in Men

Just as soy increases in endogenous estrogen effects in women, similar effects were found in men. The cross-sectional relationships of soy product intake and serum testosterone, estrone, estradiol, sex hormone-binding globulin, and dihydrotestosterone were examined in 69 Japanese men. The data suggest that soy product intake may be associated with the endogenous hormone levels in Japanese men (Nagata, Inaba, Kawakami, Kakizoe, & Shimizu, 2000).

In another study a randomized crossover dietary intervention evaluated the effects of replacing meat protein in the diet with tofu on blood concentrations of testosterone, dihydrotestosterone, androstanediol glucuronide, oestradiol, sex hormone-binding globulin (SHBG), and the free androgen index (FAI). Forty-two healthy adult males age 35 to 62 years were studied. Diets were either 150 g of lean meat or 290 g of tofu daily, providing an equivalent amount of macronutrients, with only the source of protein differing between the two diets. Each diet lasted for 4 weeks, with a 2-week interval between interventions. Urinary excretion of genistein and daidzein was significantly higher after the tofu diet. Blood concentrations of sex hormones did not differ after the two diets, but the mean testosterone:oestradiol value was 10 percent higher after the meat diet. SHBG was 3 percent higher, whereas the FAI was 7 percent lower, after the tofu diet compared with the meat diet. There was a significant correlation between the difference in SHBG and testosterone:oestradiol and weight change. Adjusting for weight change revealed SHBG to be 8.8 percent higher on the tofu diet and testosterone:oestradiol to be significantly lower. Thus, replacement of meat protein with soyabean protein, as tofu, may have a minor effect on biologically active sex hormones, which could influence prostate cancer risk. However, other factors or mechanisms may also be responsible for the different incidence rates in men on different diets (Habito, Montalto, Leslie, & Ball, 2000).

SUMMARY

Vegetarianism is experiencing a renaissance among Americans. Increasing numbers of people are eating meatless diets and seeming to thrive while doing so. However, as with most aspects of nutrition, there are cautions. Vegetarians must be careful to balance their diet to ensure adequate amounts of protein. When children and adolescents practice vegetarianism they need the counsel and guidance of a knowledgeable adult in order to avoid deficiency problems.

The use and popularity of soy products have increased dramatically during the past decade. To follow and benefit from a soy-based dietary regime, it is important to understand how to select and prepare meals to ensure proper intake of all the essential nutrients. There are many ways to buy and prepare tofu meals.

REFERENCES

Allen, M. W., Wilson, M., Ng, S. H., & Dunne, M. (2000). Values and beliefs of vegetarians and omnivores. *Journal of Social Psychology, 140*(4), 405–422.

Ball, M. J., & Ackland, M. L. (2000) Zinc intake and status in Australian vegetarians. *British Journal of Nutrition, 83*(1), 27–33.

Barnard, N. D., Scialli, A. R., Bertron, P., Hurlock, D., Edmonds, K., & Talev, L. (2000). Effectiveness of a low-fat vegetarian diet in altering serum lipids in healthy premenopausal women. *American Journal of Cardiology, 85*(8), 969–972.

Cassidy, A., Bingham, S., & Setchell, K. (1995). Biological effects of isoflavones in young women: Importance of the clinical composition of soybean products. *The British Journal of Nutrition, 74*(4), 587–601.

DeRose, D. J., Charles-Marcel, Z. L., Jamison, J. M., Muscat, J. E., Braman, M. A., McLane, G. D., & Keith Mullen, J. (2000). Vegan diet-based lifestyle program rapidly lowers homocysteine levels. *Preventive Medicine, 30*(3), 225–233.

Fraser, G. E. (1999). Diet as primordial prevention in Seventh-Day Adventists. *Preventive Medicine, 29*(6), S18–23.

Habito, R. C, Montalto, J., Leslie, E., & Ball, M. J. (2000). Effects of replacing meat with soyabean in the diet on sex hormone concentrations in healthy adult males. *British Journal of Nutrition, 84*(4), 557–563.

Kwok, T. K., Woo, J., Ho, S., & Sham, A. (2000). Vegetarianism and ischemic heart disease in older Chinese women. *Journal of the American College of Nutrition, 19*(5), 622–627.

Lamartiniere, C. A. (2000). Protection against breast cancer with genistein: A component of soy. *American Journal of Clinical Nutrition, 71*(6 Suppl.), 1705S–1707S; discussion 1708S–1709S.

Lu, L. J., Anderson, K. E., Grady, J. J., Kohen, F., & Nagamani, M. (2000). Decreased ovarian hormones during a soya diet: Implications for breast cancer prevention. *Cancer Research, 60*(15), 4112–4121.

McCarty, M. F. (1999). Vegan proteins may reduce risk of cancer, obesity, and cardiovascular disease by promoting increased glucagon activity. *Medical Hypotheses, 53*(6), 459–485.

Messina, M., & Barnes, S. (1991). The role of soy products in reducing risk of cancer. *Journal of the National Cancer Institute, 83*(8), 541–546.

Nagata, C., Inaba, S., Kawakami, N., Kakizoe, T., & Shimizu, H. (2000). Inverse association of soy product intake with serum androgen and estrogen concentrations in Japanese men. *Nutrition and Cancer, 36*(1), 14–18.

Osborne, S. (1999). Does soy have a dark side? *Natural Health* (March), 111–113, 157–158.

Rauma, A. L., & Mykkanen, H. (2000). Antioxidant status in vegetarians versus omnivores. *Nutrition, 16*(2), 111–119.

Shames, R. L., & Shames, K. H. (2001). *Thyroid power*. New York: HarperCollins.

Smith, C. F., Burke, L. E., & Wing, R. R. (2000). Vegetarian and weight-loss diets among young adults. *Obesity Research, 8*(2), 123–129.

Tikkanen, M. J., Adlercreutz, H. (2000). Dietary soy-derived isoflavone phytoestrogens. Could they have a role in coronary heart disease prevention? *Biochemical Pharmacology, 60*(1), 1–5.

van Dusseldorp, M., Schneede, J., Refsum, H., Ueland, P. M., Thomas, C. M., de Boer, E., & van Staveren, W. A. (1999). Risk of persistent cobalamin deficiency in adolescents fed a macrobiotic diet in early life. *American Journal of Clinical Nutrition, 69*(4), 664–671.

Visioli, F., Borsani, L., & Galli, C. (2000). Diet and prevention of coronary heart disease: The potential role of phytochemicals. *Cardiovascular Research, 47*(3), 419–425.

Wood, C., Cooper, D. S., Ridgway, C. (1995). *Your thyroid: A home reference,* 3rd edition. New York: Ballantine Books.

CHAPTER 15

The Joys of Juicing

WHAT IS JUICING?

Juicing is drinking fresh raw juice from fruits and vegetables. The theory of juicing is that by using the freshest fruits and vegetables we can obtain, we will have more energy and increased health and vitality. Proponents believe we will heal faster, build our immune systems, and even look younger. Anyone can juice. It is easy, quick, and may even save us money because we will eat fewer high-priced, commercially prepared, high-calorie, high-fat meals.

HOW JUICING WORKS

Within the fiber cells of every fresh fruit and vegetable are the liquids that contain the life-sustaining elements that nature provides. These elements are the carbohydrates, protein, fat, minerals, vitamins, bioflavonoids, chlorophyll, and enzymes that we need to nourish our bodies. Juice proponents contend that these life liquids lie in the most difficult part of the plant to reach, locked in the fiber of the plant, the part we call roughage. To get the full benefit of the liquids, some nutritionists think that we need to separate the liquids from the fiber. Until recently, the only way we could access these liquids was by chewing the raw vegetable or fruit.

Squeezing fruits with a hand-held tool is an alternative to eating the fruit raw, but this leaves much of the vital liquid locked in the peel. It is just not practical to hand squeeze most fruits, let alone vegetables. The alternative to chewing and squeezing is to juice the fruits and vegetables with an electric juicer. Juicing provides us with the full nutritional value of the fruits and vegetables by the masticating action of the juicer, which crushes the fibers and releases the vital liquids from the cells. The drink is pure nutritional power that can be absorbed in our bloodstreams and assimilated in every one of our 60 trillion cells within 15 minutes.

When we drink fresh vegetable and fruit juices, we are giving our bodies instant nutrition. We can feel the effects moments after consuming freshly juiced vegetables and fruits. When we eat the vegetables and fruits raw, our bodies go through an exhaustive process to extract the juice from the fiber. It is energy consuming, and it takes hours to reap these benefits. Juicing fruits and vegetables is not only a time-efficient way of getting these life liquids into our bodies, but juicing is also a very effective means of taking in large amounts of carbohydrates, minerals, vitamins, bioflavonoids, chlorophyll, and enzymes. Although we cannot eat 40 carrots or 20 apples or 12 celery stalks a day, we can juice them and consume the fruits and vegetables in a drink. This is an important aspect in the phenomenon of juicing.

Fresh fruits and vegetables are filled with nutrients and enzymes. These enzymes make the nutritional products more available to the cells by speeding their absorption. It is impossible to eat pounds and pounds of raw fruit and vegetables. For one thing, we do not have the time. For another, our systems cannot handle the roughage that would result. We do need roughage in our diets, but too much overburdens our digestive tracts. For example, how long would it take you to eat 1 pound of carrots? Probably quite a while, and it would be even longer until the nutrients were digested, absorbed, and assimilated into your body. Yet 1 pound of carrots can be juiced into one 8-ounce glass of carrot juice that we can drink in a minute. In that one glass there is enough beta-carotene to give us 20,000 to 25,000 IU of vitamin A. The RDA/DRI minimal requirement is 5,000 units. It also contains potassium, sodium, iron, phosphorous, and carbohydrates.

Remember, current recommendations are for meeting minimum daily requirements, or whatever we need to maintain borderline health. However, many nutritionists have begun to reorient their thinking to suggest optimum daily requirements. This means assessing personal daily requirements to represent the balance of vitamins, minerals, and other nutrients we need to maintain our health and lifestyles. To do this, we need to account for individual health problems as well as family history or disease-related illnesses.

Some of the recent interest in juicing has to do with results of examinations of the enormous intake of processed food by most Americans. A doughnut is a highly processed food. When you compare a doughnut to a carrot, one of the principal ingredients in health juices, you see a startling difference. Table 15–1 shows the differences between the constituents of a doughnut and a carrot.

The only thing the doughnut provides is calories, which are often not needed, and saturated fat, which most people need to avoid. The doughnut is but one example of many of the processed foods that we have become accustomed to, and for many, addicted to. Digesting processed foods is often a problem. For example, cake, bread, or the doughnut have glucose, and that glucose goes to the cells; however, glucose cannot be directly used because the body also needs minerals, vitamins, and

TABLE 15–1	Comparison of Constituents between Natural and Processed Food Product	
CONSTITUENTS	CARROT	DOUGHNUT
Glucose	Yes	Yes
Protein	Yes	No
Fats	Yes	Wrong kind; contains saturated fats
Mineral and enzymes	Yes	No
Water	Yes	No

enzymes to process the glucose. If one continues to eat only processed foods then the body has to take minerals, vitamins, and enzymes from some other parts of the body, making you weaker and more malnourished in the long run.

Juicing advocates believe that the more fresh, unprocessed foods we eat and the lower on the food chain we eat (meaning more plants), the better our immune systems will function. Eating foods in their natural state, rather than foods that have been processed, canned, or cooked, assures us of receiving the full value of the inherent life-giving substances in those foods. Juicers are quick to point out that we are the only inhabitants on this planet who cook the foods we eat. They contend that cooking severely reduces the nutritional value of foods, leaching away minerals and vitamins by cooking in water, and destroying enzymes through the action of heating.

ENZYMES

A key word for juice advocates is *enzymes*. Actually, enzymes may be the engines of life. Wherever there is life, there are enzymes. Enzymes are like catalysts. They work on a cellular level to promote chemical action without destroying, changing, or using themselves up in the process. They play a role in virtually all body activities. In fact, life could not exist without enzymes despite the presence of sufficient amounts of vitamins, minerals, and water.

Enzymes are sensitive to heat. They begin to be destroyed when exposed to temperatures above 102°F. When the temperature reaches 120°F, they die. Cooked food has no enzymes. Processed foods have no enzymes. Milk and canned juice have no enzymes. When we eat canned fruits and vegetables, we are eating food that has been exposed to high temperatures during the canning process. The government requires those high temperatures to kill bacteria, but unfortunately they also kill enzymes.

Oxygen is one of the most essential elements on earth. As soon as food is cooked, oxygen is lost and enzymes are destroyed. We cannot fully nourish the cells and tissues of our bodies with dead food. The great law of life is replenishment. If we do not eat, we die. If we do not eat the right kinds of foods to nourish our bodies, we may not only die prematurely, but we may suffer along the way.

Our bodies depend on the quality as well as the quantity of food and its compatibility with the needs of our bodies. United States citizens are the best-fed people on the planet, but we are probably the least nutritionally healthy in relation to our wealth. The point here is to begin to believe that we have the power to make ourselves well or ill according to the foods we consume. Unlike medicine, food enables us to build up or tear down the actual tissues of our bodies. When we eat right, we build strong, healthy bodies, but when diets are defective, we tear down our bodies by destroying vital tissue.

Many of us fail to realize that most healing comes from within. Nature has provided us with a wondrous immune system, but we do need to take care of it to enable our internal healing forces to function as they should. Our organs are designed to be self-repairing, but they need the raw materials of life to do their work. Juicing presents that opportunity by delivering the enzyme-rich nourishment of liquids to replenish, repair, and rejuvenate our bodies.

The theory behind fresh, raw vegetable and fruit juices is that they furnish our bodies with the necessary materials for functioning and repair, materials that are so often missing from the average diet. Even if we are not sick, we may not necessarily be healthy. Many people who appear to be in good health have borderline deficiencies, which lead to the eventual breakdown of health and the development of disease. Because of our body's miraculous tolerance, months or years may pass before we show any sign of disease.

Many maladies are the result of an incorrect diet. Constipation, folic acid anemia, chronic headaches, nervousness, and stomach trouble respond well to appropriate vegetable juices. The reason is that assimilation of the juices by the body corrects the cell chemistry composition that has become unbalanced through unnatural daily living and dieting habits. Vitality comes from food, and people who lack vitality often have decreased immunity. Deficiency of the primary elements needed in human nutrition is not only the source of most human disease, it is often the origin of mental and spiritual problems as well. People who are not vital lose their love of life.

There are other benefits as well. Apple juice has been found to inhibit human low-density lipoprotein oxidation. Dietary phenolic compounds, ubiquitous in vegetables and fruits and their juices possess antioxidant activity that have beneficial effects on human health (Pearson, Tan, German, Davis, & Gershwin, 1999).

There are six things our bodies need to stay alive, and fruits and vegetables provide all of them:

1. glucose—for energy
2. protein—for the building structure of the body

3. fats—for making hormones, which carry minerals from the blood into the digestive system

4. minerals—used for structure of the body as well as for catalysts such as enzymes, which help a chemical reaction to take place

5. vitamins—to help the body function normally (all vitamins are enzymes)

6. water—the human body is 70 percent water and it needs to be flushed and renewed daily

Raw juice therapy is a natural, drugless therapy soundly advocated by a subset of nutritionists. It is a simple and continuous practice of getting the enzymes of fruits and vegetables inside our systems. It may indeed be the secret to staying young, because with raw juice therapy, we continually revitalize ourselves.

JUICE PREPARATION

If you are interested in juicing and want to know more, there are recipe books for juices. Juicing recipes tend to fall into two groups: general daily maintenance juices and specific juices for healing.

An example of a general nutrition juice, which is available in most big-city health food bars, is carrot juice. Gather the ingredients: 5 medium carrots, 1 small apple, ½ medium beet.

Wash the carrots and remove their tops. If the apple is waxed, peel it. Remove the core. Scrub and trim the beet. Juice the ingredients and drink.

The key points to remember in preparing juices are:

1. Use the freshest fruits and vegetables that you can obtain. Grow your own if you can. The next best thing is to buy regionally grown products.

2. Buy in season.

3. Wash the produce well.

4. Peel and core fruits, with the exception of grapes and watermelons. You can use the grape peel, but discard the outer watermelon rind.

INTAKE PRINCIPLES

Juice experts advocate following four basic principles for the best use of this method:

1. When you combine two or more products, you change the chemical combination of each one so that the effect of the combination as a whole is different than taking the products individually.

2. Do not mix fruit juices with vegetable juices. The enzymes are not compatible and may cause gastritis. The exception to this principle is apple juice, which generally mixes well with other products.

3. Although you may warm your juice, do not heat it above 120°F or you will destroy the enzymes.

4. When you are ready to drink the juice, take the first mouthful slowly. In order to stimulate the salivary glands to further break down the carbohydrates, you will want to swirl the juice around in your mouth to prepare your digestive system.

I have found that sipping juices over a period of time seems more enjoyable, as well as being easier on the stomach. Remember, this is concentrated food, and your stomach will know it.

SUMMARY

Juicing is a method of vitamin, mineral, and enzyme intake that involves pulverizing fruits and vegetables into a liquid. Fiber is removed and discarded and the remaining liquid is drunk as a meal. Juice is a concentrated food that many advocate for whole body healing.

REFERENCES

Airola, P. (1991). *Juice fasting*. Sherwood, OR: Health Plus Publishers.

Calbom, C. (1999). *The juice lady's guide for juicing for health: Unleashing the power of whole fruits and vegetables*. New York: Penguin.

Crocker, P., & Eagles, S. (2000). *The juice bible*. Robert Rose.

Juicing for health, Audio Seminar (1992). Redmond, WA: Zygon International.

Keane, M. (1992). *Juicing for good health*. New York: Simon & Schuster.

Kirschner, H. E. (1957). *Live food juices*. Monrovia, CA: H.E. Kirschner Publications.

Kordich, J. (1993). *The juiceman's power of juicing*. New York: Warner Books.

Null, G., and Null, S. (1992). *The joy of juicing recipe guide: Creative cooking with your juicer*. New York: Avery.

Pearson, D. A, Tan, C. H., German, J. B., Davis, P. A., & Gershwin, M. E. (1999). Apple juice inhibits human low density lipoprotein oxidation. *Life Science, 64*(21), 1913–1920.

Rodnitzky, D. (2000). *Ultimate juicing: Delicious recipes for over 125 of the best fruits and vegetables combinations*. Schoolcraft, MI: Prima Communications.

Walker, N. W. (1970). *Fresh vegetable and fruit juices*. Prescott, AZ: Norwalk Press.

CHAPTER 16

The Healing Powers of Wine

The range and power of modern pharmaceutical agents have given healers new resources to treat infections, soothe chronic pain, and prevent infectious diseases. Yet, despite these technological advances, wine remains one of the safest, easiest to make, and one of the most restorative natural substances on Earth.

Wine differs from most other medicinal agents in that it can also be regarded as a food. It meets the two basic dietary requirements: it provides energy, and it contributes to the maintenance of the body.

When we begin to use wine as a healing food, we can draw with some degree of comfort on intelligent observation and experience recorded over a period of several thousands of years. In addition, we can buttress that lengthy experience with a substantial volume of modern scientific investigation.

WINE USED SENSIBLY

Before addressing the beneficial and medicinal uses of wine, let me first say that it is imperative that this substance be used in moderation and with good judgment. As we all know, there are those who cannot control their intake of alcoholic drinks. Whether this is a genetic trait or a learned behavior is debatable, but the facts are that many people who begin to drink continue to do so until they are either drunk or develop a high tolerance for alcohol intake. According to the U.S. government's National Institute on Alcohol Abuse and Alcoholism, roughly 1 in 7 of the nation's 100 million drinkers has alcohol-related health problems. Knowing these facts should alert us to the potential deleterious effects of this substance.

Certainly, wine should be avoided whenever consumption would put the individual or others at risk. This includes times of pregnancy and when driving.

Wine, like herbs, must be used with knowledge and with caution. It is not a substance to be abused, but one to use with conscious choice and for purposes of relaxation or medicinal applications.

WINE AS A FOOD

Wine is an alcoholic beverage made from fermented grape juice. Wines are colored red, white, or rosé and are labeled as dry, medium, or sweet. They fall into three basic categories: natural or "table" wines, which have an alcohol content of 8 to 14 percent; sparkling wines, such as champagne, which have an alcohol content similar to table wines and which contain carbon dioxide; and fortified wines, which have an alcohol content of 15 to 24 percent, and are drunk either as aperitifs or with dessert, depending on their sweetness. The various types of fortified wines include sherry, port, and aromatic wines and bitters such as vermouth.

Traditionally, we serve wine at the table where it is used as a food along with other foods. Because of the presence of organic acids, tannins, and other components, our bodies absorb the alcohol in wine much more slowly than the alcohol in other alcoholic solutions. We usually sip wine with our meals, resulting in still slower absorption of the alcohol, yielding relatively low and safe blood-alcohol concentrations.

Red wine should be served at room temperature, while white and rosé wines should be chilled prior to drinking. An Oriental version of wine, sake (pronounced sah'-kee), is a sweet and colorless fermented wine. Often called Japanese rice wine, it has a high alcoholic content (12 to 16 percent by volume) and none of the carbon dioxide found in other fermented drinks such as beer. Sake is made from rice that is cleaned, steamed, treated with a special yeast, and allowed to ferment for 4 to 5 weeks. Near the end of the fermentation, more rice and water are added, and a second fermentation takes place. The resulting liquor is drawn off, filtered, and placed in casks for maturing. It is served warm in a small table container, poured into thimble-size cups and sipped. Table 16–1 details the calorie content of major wine types, while Table 16–2 details some wine food facts.

WINE AS AN ENERGY SOURCE

Wine supplies useful energy, mostly from alcohol, at the rate of approximately 7 calories per gram, and from carbohydrates, at the rate of 4 calories per gram. Table wines average about 80 calories per 100 cc or 24 calories per ounce, while cocktail and dessert wines average about 150 calories per 100 cc or 45 calories per ounce.

TABLE 16–1 Calorie Content of Major Wine Types

WINE	CAL/100 CC.	CAL/OZ.	SERVING (OZ.)	CAL/TYPICAL SERVING
Red Table Wines				
Burgundy	80.2	24.1	4	96.4
Cabernet	82.8	24.8	4	99.2
Chianti	81.8	24.5	4	98.0
Claret	79.8	23.9	4	95.6
Zinfandel	81.8	23.5	4	94.0
Rosé Table Wines	78.3	23.5	4	94.0
White Table Wines				
Chablis	73.8	22.1	4	88.4
Champagne	82.5	24.8	4	99.2
Rhine	76.7	23.0	4	92.0
Riesling	74.8	22.4	4	89.6
Dry sauterne	74.8	23.2	4	89.6
Sauterne	77.2	23.2	4	92.8
Sweet sauterne	87.1	26.1	4	104.4
Cocktail and Dessert Wines				
Red port	161.3	48.4	2	96.8
White port	150.0	45.0	2	90.0
Muscatel	163.2	49.0	2	98.0
Dry sherry	130.1	39.0	2	78.0
Sweet sherry	152.7	45.8	2	91.6
Dry vermouth	113.2	34.0	2	102.0
Sweet vermouth	150.4	45.1	2	135.3

TABLE 16–2 Wine Food Facts

1. Wine is technically a food, a source of energy for work and body maintenance.

2. In moderate quantities, wine has no deleterious effect on growth or development, but it is not recommended during pregnancy.

3. The content of B vitamins and minerals in wine make it a desirable supplemental source of these substances in daily diets.

4. Most wines may be effectively incorporated into low-sodium diets.

5. Wine resembles gastric juice more closely than does any other natural beverage.

6. In moderate amounts, wine stimulates gastric secretion and motility, increases bile flow, and assists the natural processes of evacuation of the colon.

CASE STUDY: Agnes

Agnes was 32 years old. She had been divorced for two years and was conspicuously underweight. It seemed no matter how she tried, Agnes could not muster the desire to eat. Six months ago, she quit her job and went back home to Mississippi to live with her parents. They tried to help her shake her depression and helped care for her 10-year-old son. They made every attempt to entice their daughter to eat their pancake and bacon breakfasts and old-fashioned meat and potato dinners. Despite their best efforts, Agnes had no appetite. She simply would not eat. All she did was mope around the house sipping glass after glass of iced tea and feeling sorry for herself.

Two weeks after Agnes had moved back with her parents, a neighbor invited her to visit. During the visit, she was offered a glass of sherry. She accepted it and found that the salutary effects caused her to stay longer than she had intended. She even indulged in a plate of sandwiches that her hostess offered during their enjoyable visit. They had so much fun that Agnes agreed to return to pick up where they left off.

When she returned, she once again accepted a glass of sherry. To her surprise, not only did she eat the plate of sandwiches but also accepted and enjoyed a piece of carrot cake. She returned home happy, satisfied, and full. In fact, she got along with the neighbor so well that they decided to make a biweekly routine of their afternoon rendezvous. The next week Agnes discovered that the Tuesday and Friday visits were the highlight of her week. She felt like she had met someone with whom she had something in common, and after each visit, she returned home feeling relaxed and full.

Within 2 weeks, she began to make a correlation between the sherry and her appetite, so she decided to try the experiment at home with her dad. Sure enough, it seemed to make a difference. She soon accepted the fact that with a glass of sherry before meals, she relaxed more, stopped thinking about her miserable situation, and actually had an appetite for dinner. At the same time, she decided to follow her mother's advice and stop drinking the iced tea all afternoon. Within a month's time, her anorexia abated and she began putting on some much needed weight.

Observation

In people suffering from anorexia and/or loss of weight, wine intake has a double beneficial effect: calorie intake and relaxation. Goetzl (1953) reported on a series of patients whose average caloric intake was

(Continued on next page)

increased by 60 percent over a 3-month period, accompanied by a 12 per-cent increase in body weight. Wine stimulates the appetite directly through its physiological effect on the buccal mucosa. Based on laboratory studies, the wine components of acetic, tartaric, and tannic acids have been reported to have a specific appetite-stimulating action (Irvin, Ahokas, & Goetzl, 1950). In general, relatively small amounts of wine preceding and during mealtimes stimulate the appetite by physiological as well as psy-chological means (Dufour, Archer, & Gordis, 1992). However, ingestion of larger quantities, especially during a prolonged period before meals, may depress the appetite and promote drinking rather than eating. Appetite stimulation and relaxation are, of course, the goal for people like Agnes.

USE IN WEIGHT REDUCTION

Wine can also play a role in the control of obesity, especially when emotional tension is a contributory factor in the overeating. For many of us, a reducing diet is easy to come by, easy to understand, but extremely difficult to follow. Lolli's stud-ies have shown that the appropriate use of wine can contribute to a weight reduc-tion program by making it easier for us to adhere to a prescribed diet. Amounts proposed for this purpose range from 6 to 8 ounces of dry wine, taken approxi-mately half an hour before the major meal of the day. Use before bedtime may reduce insomnia, lessening the craving for a bedtime snack (Balboni, 1963). When a dry wine was incorporated into a reducing diet, investigators demonstrated that most subjects naturally decreased their carbohydrate intake (Lolli, 1963).

MEDICINAL USE IN ILLNESS AND DISEASE

It is interesting to note that there is scant reference regarding the medicinal use of wine from 1960 to 1990. Reference to wine or alcohol in the journals during the past three decades has focused on alcohol addiction and its treatment. Hence, many of us have not been exposed to the beneficial effects of this food. Only since 1990 have we begun to see a resurgence in published reports regarding the bene-fits of wine.

Emotional Tension

The most obvious site of action of wine is in the central nervous system. We need not be skilled in psychology to note the effects of moderate quantities of wine at social gatherings. The speech and bearing of people and the play of features bear witness to its power. Restraints are removed, overly acute sensibilities are blunted, and little excitabilities are smoothed. Ideas and mental images follow each other with greater rapidity. A "cerebral sense of richness" occurs and lastly, a condition of euphoria and a more serene state of consciousness ensues. This statement, which may have been made by any observer today was, in fact, made more than 90 years ago (Billings, 1903). In slightly different forms, it has been made by others 600 years ago and even several millennia ago (Lucia, 1963).

Coronary Heart Disease

The heart is a primary focal area for the medicinal use of wine. Relief from anginal pain with wine, cordials, and brandy has been regularly reported since the observations of Heberden (1786) in the 18th century. When health care providers worked with angina patients during the 1950s, alcoholic beverages ranked second only to nitrates in controlling this symptom (White, 1951). I remember well working evenings on the medical wards in a large hospital in New York City during the late 1960s and passing out many 2-ounce cups of brandy or sherry to our cardiac patients. We routinely kept the bottles in the medicine cabinet with the other generic medications. Remember, those were the days before unit dose and pharmacy preparation of medications. Looking at this from within the framework of a lifetime, it was not so long ago. But the fact of the matter is, it worked. It was inexpensive and easy to dispense. Patients not only got the vasodilation effect but also seemed to relax and sleep better.

Current literature is less romantic and more factual. The relationship between alcohol consumption and angiographically documented coronary artery disease was examined among 484 men who underwent coronary arteriography. A decrease in the average coronary artery disease scores was observed with increasing alcohol consumption until a mean consumption of about 100 ml per day. These findings provide additional evidence that the reduction of the clinical coronary risk observed in moderate alcohol consumers might be secondary, at least partly, to an anatomically less extensive disease (Ducimetiere et al., 1993).

The French Paradox

Epidemiological studies suggest that the consumption of wine, particularly of red wine, reduces the incidence of mortality and morbidity from coronary heart disease. This has given rise to what is now popularly termed the *French paradox,* the apparent compatibility of a high-fat diet with a low incidence of coronary atherosclerosis. The cardioprotective effect has been attributed to antioxidants present in the polyphenol fraction of red wine. Grapes contain a variety of antioxidants, including resveratrol, catechin, epicatechin, and proanthocyanidins. Of these, resveratrol is present mainly in grape skin while proanthocyanidin is present in the seeds. There is evidence that red wine extract as well as resveratrol and proanthocyanidins are equally effective in reducing myocardial ischemic reperfusion injury, which suggests that these red wine polyphenolic antioxidants play a crucial role in cardioprotection (Das et al., 1999).

The French paradox has been attributed to the regular drinking of red wine. However, the alcohol content of wine may not be the sole explanation for this protection. Red wine contains phenolic compounds, and the antioxidant properties of these may have an important role. In in vitro studies with phenolic substances in red wine and normal human low-density lipoprotein (LDL), researchers found that red wine inhibits the copper-catalyses oxidation of LDL. Wine diluted 1,000-fold and containing 10 millimoles/L total phenolics inhibited LDL oxidation significantly more than alpha-tocopherol. The findings show that the nonalcoholic components of red wine have potent antioxidant properties toward oxidation of human LDL (Frankel et al., 1993; "Inhibition of LDL," 1993).

Studies indicate that the consumption of alcohol at the level of intake in France (20 to 30 grams per day or two to three 4-ounce servings per day) can reduce the risk of coronary heart disease (CHD) by at least 40 percent. Alcohol is believed to protect from CHD by preventing atherosclerosis through the action of high-density-lipoprotein cholesterol; but serum concentrations of this factor are no higher in France than in other countries. Reexamination of previous results suggests that moderate alcohol intake does not prevent CHD through an effect on atherosclerosis, but rather through a hemostatic mechanism. Data from Wales show that platelet aggregation, which is related to CHD, is inhibited significantly by alcohol at levels of intake associated with reduced risk of CHD. Inhibition of platelet reactivity by wine may be one explanation for protection from CHD in France, since pilot studies have shown that platelet reactivity is lower in France than in Scotland (Renaud, 1992).

Contemporary Research Studies

Recently there has been an abundant amount of new research that validates the potential benefits of wine. Several studies are summarized here.

EFFECTS OF DIFFERENT TYPES OF ALCOHOLIC BEVERAGES ON MYOCARDIAL INFARCTION

Wine may be more beneficial for the heart than other types of alcoholic beverages. One research study assessed the relationship between myocardial infarction (MI) and consumption of different types of alcoholic beverages, both low doses (1 to 4 drinks a day), and high doses (more than 4 drinks a day.) The researchers found that:

- small doses (1 to 4 drinks a day) of alcohol are associated with a slightly reduced risk of mortality and CHD.
- small doses of wine, beer, and spirits are equally beneficial.
- apart from a direct beneficial effect of low doses of alcohol on mortality and CHD, some psychological factors may contribute to its beneficial effect.
- high doses (5 or more drinks a day) of alcohol are not associated with a reduced risk of death and CHD.
- apart from a direct effect of alcohol, confounding factors, particularly those of a psychological nature, may well contribute to the loss of benefits (Cleophas, 1999).

EFFECTS OF MODERATE CONSUMPTION OF ALCOHOL IN COMPARISON WITH MINERAL WATER

Moderate consumption of red wine, beer, and spirits is associated with a reduced risk of CHD. Part of this inverse association may be explained by its effects on high-density lipoproteins (HDL). Paraoxonase, an HDL-associated enzyme, has been suggested to protect against LDL oxidation. Researchers examined the effects of moderate consumption of red wine, beer, and spirits in comparison with mineral water on paraoxonase activity in serum. In a diet-controlled, randomized, crossover study, 11 healthy middle-age men consumed four glasses of red wine, beer, or spirits with evening dinner for 3 weeks. The control group drank four glasses of water. At the end of each 3-week period, blood samples were collected pre- and postprandially and after an overnight fast. Fasting paraoxonase activity was higher after intake of wine and spirits than after water consumption, but did not differ significantly between the three alcoholic beverages. Similar effects were observed pre- and postprandially. The increases in paraoxonase activity were strongly correlated with coincident increases in concentrations of HDL-C and apo A-I. These data suggest that increased serum paraoxonase may be one of the biological mechanisms underlying the reduced CHD risk in moderate alcohol consumers (van der Gaag et al., 1999).

The consumption of red wine has been reported to impart a greater benefit in the prevention of CHD than the consumption of other alcoholic beverages. Epidemiological studies have demonstrated an inverse correlation between moderate wine and alcohol consumption and morbidity and mortality from CHD. This protective effect has been associated with an increase in the plasma level of HDL-cholesterol, as it is well known that plasma HDL is inversely correlated with CHD. In addition, it has become evident that blood platelets contribute to the rate of development of atherosclerosis and CHD through several mechanisms (Ruf, 1999).

Recent studies have shown HDL-cholesterol levels can explain only 50 percent of the protective effect of alcoholic beverages. The other 50 percent may be partly related to decreased platelet activity. The antiplatelet activity of wine is explained not only by ethanol but also by the polyphenolic components with which red wines are richly endowed. Several studies carried out in humans and animals have shown that wine phenolics could exert their effects by reducing prostanoid synthesis from arachidonate. In addition, it has been suggested that wine phenolics could reduce platelet activity mediated by nitric oxide. Moreover, wine phenolics increase vitamin E levels while decreasing the oxidation of platelets submitted to oxidative stress. However, a rebound phenomenon of hyperaggregability is observed after acute alcohol consumption but not after wine consumption. This protection afforded by wine has been duplicated in animals with grape phenolics added to alcohol. This rebound phenomenon could explain ischemic strokes or sudden deaths known to occur after episodes of drunkenness. It appears that wine and wine phenolics in particular could significantly inhibit platelet aggregation and that this could explain, at least in part, the protective effect of red wine against atherosclerosis and coronary heart disease (Ruf, 1999).

BOTH RED WINE EXTRACT AND TRANSRESVERTROL ARE EQUALLY CARDIOPROTECTIVE

The beneficial effect of red wine is increasingly being attributed to certain antioxidants comprising the polyphenol fraction of red wine such as transresveratrol. The results of one study indicate that resveratrol possesses cardioprotective effects which may be attributed to its peroxyl radical scavenging activity (Ray et al., 1999).

In another study, the cardioprotective action of red wine was measured by preperfusing isolated rat hearts with ethanol-free red wine extract for 15 minutes before subjecting them to 30 minutes of global ischemia followed by 2 hours of reperfusion. Results of this study demonstrated that both red wine extract and transresveratrol were equally cardioprotective, as evidenced by their abilities to improve postischemic ventricular functions including developed pressure and aortic flow. These compounds also reduced myocardial infarct size compared with the control hearts. The ethanol-treated group displayed slightly better functional recovery, which deteriorated sharply toward the end of the reperfusion period, and the extent of infarction was comparable to that of the control group. Taken together, the results of this study indicate that red wines are cardioprotective by their ability to function as an in vivo antioxidant (Sato et al., 2000).

THE RELATION BETWEEN INTAKE OF DIFFERENT TYPES OF ALCOHOL AND DEATH FROM ALL CAUSES

A study examined the relation between intake of different types of alcohol and death from all causes, CHD, and cancer in 13,064 men and 11,459 women 20 to 98 years old. Compared with nondrinkers, light drinkers who avoided wine had a relative risk for death from all causes and those who drank wine had a relative risk. Heavy drinkers who avoided wine were at higher risk for death from all causes than were heavy drinkers who included wine in their alcohol intake. Wine drinkers had significantly lower mortality from both coronary heart disease and cancer than did nonwine drinkers. Thus, wine intake may have a beneficial effect on all-cause mortality that is additive to that of alcohol. This effect may be attributable to a reduction in death from both CHD and cancer (Gronbaek et al., 2000).

PURPLE GRAPE JUICE AND CORONARY ARTERY DISEASE

There is increasing evidence to indicate that the cardioprotective effects of red wine consumption are attributed to certain polyphenolic constituents of grapes (Sato, Maulik, Ray, Bagchi, & Das, 1999). Results of one study showed that grape seed-proanthocyanidins possess a cardioprotective effect against ischemia reperfusion injury. Such cardioprotective property, at least in part, may be attributed to its ability to directly scavenge peroxyl and hydroxyl radicals and to reduce oxidative stress developed during ischemia and reperfusion (Sato et al., 1999).

In vitro, the flavonoid components of red wine and purple grape juice are powerful antioxidants that induce endothelium-dependent vasodilation of vascular rings derived from rat aortas and human coronary arteries. Although improved endothelial function and inhibition of LDL oxidation may be potential mechanisms by which red wine and flavonoids reduce cardiovascular risk, the in vivo effects of grape products on endothelial function and LDL oxidation had not been investigated. A specific study assessed the effects of ingesting purple grape juice on endothelial function and LDL susceptibility to oxidation in patients with coronary artery disease (CAD). That study found that short-term ingestion of purple grape juice reduces LDL susceptibility to oxidation in CAD patients. Improved endothelium-dependent vasodilation and prevention of LDL oxidation are potential mechanisms by which flavonoids in purple grape products may prevent cardiovascular events, independent of alcohol content (Stein, Keevil, Wiebe, Aeschlimann, & Folts, 1999).

Other Conditions

During our lifetime, wine has been found to be beneficial in a host of other conditions. These include renal disease, infectious diseases, Parkinsonism, gout, and viral hepatitis. However, even though we know that wine does have beneficial effects, some cautions are advisable. First, we all know the potentially deadly effects of overconsumption and addiction. All kinds of alcohol addiction programs and support groups have arisen over the past three decades to combat alcohol abuse. The caution with wine, as with most other areas of life, is to use it in moderation. Too much can be detrimental.

The second caution relates to women. Recent studies report a positive correlation between alcohol consumption and breast cancer. A United States Nurses' Health Study in 1986 examined alcohol consumption in relation to risk of breast cancer via dietary questionnaires that were administered both before and after diagnosis. Analysis of the data demonstrated an elevated risk of breast cancer among women who drank 30 grams or more of alcohol daily (about two drinks) as compared to nondrinkers (Giovannucci et al., 1993). In another questionnaire study done in Spain, data suggested that even at moderate levels of alcohol intake (less than 8 grams per day), a 50 percent increase in risk of breast cancer was found. Consumption of 20 grams or more of alcohol per day was associated with a 70 percent elevation in breast cancer risk compared with that of nondrinkers (Martin-Moreno, 1993). The significant thing to note in both of these studies, however, is that no differentiation was made regarding the kind of alcohol consumed. Alcohols in beverages such as bourbon, scotch, and rum are of a different substance and potency than the alcohol in wines.

The differences among the types of alcohol become apparent upon analysis. In a study of age-specific consumption of beer, wine, and liquor and the occurrence of disease, the findings were noteworthy. Overall, there was a modest indication that high levels of alcohol consumption (11 or more drinks per week) were associated with increased risk of large bowel cancer. In site-specific analyses, only rectal cancer demonstrated a significant linear trend with increasing consumption. Beer was associated significantly with rectal cancer. Wine consumption was associated inversely with rectal cancers. These relationships appeared to be consistent for recent, past, and total lifetime consumption and were not attributable to differences in dietary habits (Newcomb, Storer, & Marcus, 1993). Again, care must be taken to differentiate between not only the amount, but the type of alcohol consumed.

Potential Deleterious Effects

Wine has beneficial and harmful effects on health at the same time (Cleophas, 1999). There is a well-established correlation between alcohol consumption and mental impairment. Figure 16–1 details blood alcohol levels and areas of impairment.

Besides mental impairment, overconsumption of alcohol products, primarily wine, may have other deleterious effects. Most wines have a significant amount of sulfites, used as a preservative, which in some people can trigger adverse reactions such as asthma, migraine headaches, and other problems. American wines, for the most part, tend to have a higher concentration of these preservatives than their European counterparts. For those people who realize they are sensitive, they can seek wines produced without preservatives. These products are sometimes sold in health food stores.

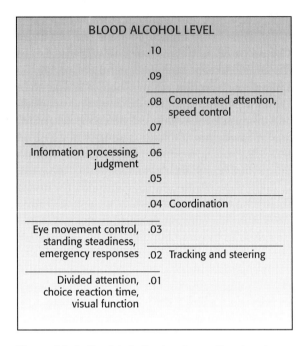

Figure 16–1   Blood alcohol levels and areas of impairment.
Source: National Highway Traffic Safety Administration (NHTSA).

SUMMARY

Table wines have been with us since time immemorial. Wine is a food that when consumed in moderation can be beneficial as a relaxant or as a stimulant, depending upon the setting and the type of wine ingested. Some people like to think of wine as a fruited beverage because it is derived from grapes. Wine may be used as a healing food when taken with a sense of consciousness and care.

There was an interest in wine for medicinal purposes in antiquity; it arose again in the 1950s when, for example, wine was suggested as an aid for anorexia. Interestingly, there were only scant reports of its beneficial effects until the late 1990s. At that time the positive effects of the French paradox were noted and research on the medicinal effects of wine was renewed. The beneficial effect of red wine is increasingly being attributed to certain antioxidants comprising the polyphenol fraction of red wine such as transresveratrol and the flavonoid components of both red wine and purple grape juice.

It is important to note that overconsumption of wine is deleterious to health, and therefore people need to be disciplined with their intake. As with most things, moderation is the key.

REFERENCES

Balboni, C. (1963). Alcohol in relation to dietary patterns. In S. P. Lucia (Ed.), *Alcohol and civilization*. New York: McGraw-Hill.

Billings, J. S., et al. (1903). *Physiological aspects of liquor problems*. New York: Houghton Mifflin.

Cleophas, T. J. (1999). Wine, beer and spirits and the risk of myocardial infarction: A systematic review. *Biomedical Pharmacotherapy, 53*(9), 417–423.

Das, D. K., Sato, M., Ray, P. S., Maulik, G., Engelman, R. M., Bertelli, A. A., & Bertelli, A. (1999). Cardioprotection of red wine: Role of polyphenolic antioxidants. *Drugs Under Experimental and Clinical Research, 25*(2–3), 115–120.

Ducimetiere, P., Guize, L., Marciniak, A., Milton, H., Richard, J., & Rufat, P. (1993). Arteriographically documented coronary artery disease and alcohol consumption in French men. *European Heart Journal, 14*(6), 727–733.

Dufour M. C., Archer L., & Gordis, E. (1992). Alcohol and the elderly. *Clinical Geriatric Medicine, 8*(1), 127–141.

Frankel, E. N., Kanner, J., German, J. B., Parks, E., & Kinsella, J. E. (1993). Inhibition of oxidation of human low-density lipoprotein by phenolic substances in red wine. *Lancet, 341,* 454–457.

Giovannucci, E., et al. (1993). Recall and selection bias in reporting past alcohol consumption. *Cancer Causes Control, 4*(5), 441–448.

Goetzl, F. R. (1953). *A note on the possible usefulness of wine in the management of anorexia*. Oakland, CA: Permanente Foundation.

Gronbaek, M., Becker, U., Johansen, D., Gottschau, A., Schnohr, P., Hein, H. O., Jensen, G., & Sorensen, T. I. (2000). Type of alcohol consumed and mortality from all causes, coronary heart disease, and cancer. *Annals of Internal Medicine, 133*(6), 411–419.

Heberden, W. (1786). Some account of a disorder of the breast. *Medical transcriptions of the Royal College of Physicians in London, 2,* 59–67.

Inhibition of LDL oxidation by phenolic substances in red wine: A clue to the French paradox? (1993). *Nutrition Review, 51*(6), 185–187.

Irvin, D. L., Ahokas, A. J., & Goetzl, F. R. (1950). The influence of ethyl alcohol in low concentrations upon olfactory acuity and the sensation complex of appetite and satiety. *Permanente Foundation Medical Bulletin, 8,* 97–101.

Lolli, G. (1963). The role of wine in the treatment of obesity. *New York State Journal of Medicine, 62,* 3438–3443.

Lolli, G., Serianni, E., Golder, G., Mariani, A., & Toner, M. (1952). Relationships between intake of carbohydrate-rich foods and intake of wine and other alcoholic beverages. *Quarterly Journal Studies Alcohol, 13,* 401–420.

Lucia, S. P. (1963). The antiquity of alcohol in diet and medicine. In S. P. Lucia (Ed.), *Alcohol and civilization*. New York: McGraw-Hill.

Martin-Moreno, J., et al. (1993). Alcoholic beverage consumption and risk of breast cancer in Spain. *Cancer Causes Control, 4*(4), 345–353.

Newcomb, P., Storer, B., & Marcus, P. (1993). Cancer of the large bowel in women in relation to alcohol consumption: A case control study in Wisconsin. *Cancer Causes Control, 4*(5), 405–411.

Ray, P. S., Maulik, G., Cordis, G. A., Bertelli, A. A., Bertelli, A., & Das, D. K. (1999). The red wine antioxidant resveratrol protects isolated rat hearts from ischemia reperfusion injury. *Free Radical Biological Medicine, 27*(1–2), 160–169.

Renaud, S. (1992). Wine, alcohol, platelets, and the French paradox for coronary heart disease. *Lancet, 339,* 1523–1526.

Ruf, J. C. (1999). Wine and polyphenols related to platelet aggregation and atherothrombosis. *Drugs Under Experimental and Clinical Research, 25*(2–3), 125–131.

Sato, M., Maulik, G., Ray, P. S., Bagchi, D., & Das, D. K. (1999). Cardioprotective effects of grape seed proanthocyanidin against ischemic reperfusion injury. *Journal of Molecular and Cellular Cardiology, 31*(6), 1289–1297.

Sato, M., Ray, P. S., Maulik, G., Maulik, N., Engelman, R. M., Bertelli, A. A., Bertelli, A., & Das, D. K. (2000). Myocardial protection with red wine extract. *Journal of Cardiovascular Pharmacology, 35*(2), 263–268.

Stein, J. H., Keevil, J. G., Wiebe, D. A., Aeschlimann, S., & Folts, J. D. (1999). Purple grape juice improves endothelial function and reduces the susceptibility of LDL cholesterol to oxidation in patients with coronary artery disease. *Circulation, 100*(10), 1050–1055.

van der Gaag, M. S., van Tol, A., Scheek, L. M., James, R. W., Urgert, R., Schaafsma, G., & Hendriks, H. F. (1999) Daily moderate alcohol consumption increases serum paraoxonase activity: A diet-controlled, randomised intervention study in middle-aged men. *Atherosclerosis, 147*(2), 405–410.

White, P. D. (1951). *Heart disease.* New York: Macmillan.

CHAPTER
17

Controversies in Nutrition

THE NATURE OF CONTROVERSY

Controversy is not new, the pros and cons of nutritional issues have been debated throughout history. History is full of examples of public health, commerce, and politics in conflict. Sometimes, insufficient attention is given to a controversy. Let's look at the United Kingdom (UK), for an example: In recent years attempts to protect UK egg producers, after the discovery of *Salmonella enteritidis* in hens' eggs, strained previously good working relationships between medical and veterinary epidemiologists and ended the political career of a government minister who spoke out in defense of the public health. Against the background lessons of earlier high-profile public health problems in the UK, conflict should have been avoided when bovine spongiform encephalopathy (BSE or Mad Cow Disease) started. We might have expected that BSE's public health implications would be recognized and researched earlier, and that public announcements would be timely and clear. Unfortunately this was not the case and, in the opinion of some, it looks as though similar mistakes will be repeated over genetically modified foods (O'Brien, 2000) and other controversial food issues.

Each of the following areas of nutrition can be classified as controversial. Despite the widespread approval of these issues by some caregivers, others continue to be skeptical.

MEGAVITAMIN THERAPY

Megavitamin therapy is the name of a controversial mode of nutrient therapy that involves the ingestion of large doses of vitamins. Linus Pauling was the first to use the term *orthomolecular* to characterize the treatment of human disease with nutrients that naturally occur in the human body. The basic premise of orthomolecular medicine is that the greatest long-term health benefits in disease treatment are derived from establishing the concentration of essential nutrients in the body. This is done by adjusting diets, eliminating junk foods, and, most controversially, ingesting large (mega) doses of various nutrients. Pauling became best known when he advocated megadoses of vitamin C for treatment of the common cold.

Orthomolecular medicine is primarily utilized in the treatment of psychiatric disorders. Initially used to treat schizophrenia, the scope of disorders thought to improve with the application of orthomolecular principles has continually broadened. It includes, for example, epilepsy, autism, senility, arthritis, and allergies. Orthomolecular therapy is also used to treat diseases and chronic problems such as backaches and psoriasis.

While treatment programs vary, the main focus is on megavitamin therapy followed by a combination of other essential nutrients that are lacking or inadequate in the body. Drugs are used infrequently, the goal being to subsist on nutrients alone. Treatment programs are developed through clinical tests, psychiatric examinations, and consultation to identify the different nutrient requirements of each patient. Some believe, although this is highly controversial, that awareness of drug side effects and the desire for natural treatments will make orthomolecular medicine a dominant therapeutic tool of the future.

The controversy over megavitamin therapy arises from conflicting research as to its effectiveness. For example, a study was done to assess the efficacy of adjunctive megavitamin and dietary treatment in schizophrenia. A random allocation double-blind, controlled comparison of dietary supplement and megavitamin treatment, and an alternative procedure was given for 5 months to 19 outpatients diagnosed with schizophrenia. In addition to usual follow-up, the experimental group received amounts of megavitamins based on their individual serum vitamin levels. The control group received 25 mg of vitamin C. Five months of treatment showed marked differences in serum levels of vitamins but no consistent self-reported symptomatic or behavioral differences between groups. This study does not provide evidence supporting a positive relationship between regulation of levels of serum vitamins and clinical outcome in schizophrenia (Vaughan & McConaghy, 1999).

FOOD ADDITIVES

A food additive is a nonfood substance added to food during processing to preserve or improve its color, texture, flavor, or value. By definition, the nonfood class also includes substances that may indirectly become components of food. For example, a chemical used to make cereal packaging paper is considered a food additive if the packaged cereal absorbs even minute quantities of the additive.

Iron, minerals, and vitamins are regularly introduced into foods to compensate for losses during processing or to provide additional nutrients. Iodine may be added to salt, vitamin A to margarine, and vitamin D to milk. Flavoring agents, including salts, spices, essential oils, and natural and synthetic flavors, make up the largest single class of additives. Additives that improve texture include emulsifiers, stabilizers, and thickeners. Gums, dextrins, and starches are used to give more substance to soups and desserts. Pectin and gelatin are added to thicken jams and jellies. Lecithin is the primary emulsifier used in salad dressings and chocolates.

The additives used to preserve food are primarily chemical antimicrobial agents such as the benzoates, propionates, and sorbates that retard spoilage caused by bacteria, yeasts, and molds. Antioxidants are used to keep fats and oils from spoiling and to prevent discoloration of smoked or canned meats. Ascorbic acid is used to prevent the discoloration of canned fruits.

The wide use of synthetic additives is a 20th-century phenomenon associated with the growth of the food industry. Some of the additives used today are labeled in the terminology of the U.S. Food and Drug Administration (FDA) as *generally recognized as safe* (GRAS). A number of these substances had been used before 1958 when amendments to the Food, Drug, and Cosmetic Act required that new food additives be tested for safety with no recorded evidence of harmful effects. Others were given GRAS status after 1958. Synthetic food colors have also come under FDA scrutiny, and some dyes are now prohibited as food additives. In 1986 the FDA banned sulfites for use as color preservatives in fresh fruits and vegetables. The FDA had previously required labeling of sulfite contents in other foods.

Concern is also growing about chemicals that indirectly find their way into foods by way of pesticide residues on fruits and vegetables or through medications and stimulants given to animals. In 1979 the FDA banned the use of the synthetic hormone diethylstilbestrol in cattle because residues were showing up in meat products. In the early 1990s, the FDA and other federal agencies responsible for food safety increased the amount of testing being performed for pesticides.

ORGANICALLY GROWN FOODS

Organically grown foods are foods that are grown without the use of chemical fertilizers or pesticides. Natural foods are usually thought of as foods processed without chemical additives.

Interest in organically grown foods has developed rapidly in the United States since studies in the 1960s linked certain food additives with cancer and other diseases. It is widely acknowledged that some pesticides used on crops and some chemicals used in food processing may be harmful to our health. However, for many chemicals, health hazards have not been proved, nor has it been proved that organically grown foods are nutritionally superior to those grown using chemical fertilizers.

Organic health foods and the claims about their benefits are among the more controversial and complex issues being debated by food regulators. Proponents state that organic foods may reduce health care expenditures and believe that their health claims are a legitimate nutrition education tool that informs consumers. Opponents respond that it is the total diet that is important for health. Moreover, they argue that health claims will enable manufacturers to indulge in marketing hyperbole and essentially blur the distinction between food and drugs. There is a need to maintain a general prohibition on health claims while accommodating specific exemptions supported by scientific substantiation (Lawrence & Rayner, 1998).

FOOD IRRADIATION

Recent well-publicized outbreaks of food-borne illness have heightened general interest in food safety. Food irradiation is a technology that has been approved for use in selected foods in the United States since 1963. Widespread use of irradiation remains controversial, however, because of public concern regarding the safety of the technology and the wholesomeness of irradiated foods (Shea, 2000).

After 40 years of experimentation and controversy over the nutritional and environmental safety implications of preserving and disinfecting foods with radioactive materials, food irradiation has become a reality. Essentially, food irradiation is a process in which food is exposed to gamma radiation from radioactive materials such as cobalt 60 or cesium-137 or through linear accelerator electron beams to kill bacteria, insects, or parasites that may be present.

Although the doses used on food are too weak to actually make the food radioactive, they are strong enough to disrupt the chemical bonds that hold molecules together, thus killing or inhibiting the growth of organisms that cause disease, spoilage, and other forms of deterioration. A typical chest X-ray delivers a dose of 1/100 of 1 rad (radiation absorbed dose). In contrast, the amount of energy used in food irradiation, measured in units called *Grays,* is considerably higher—100,000 rads = 1,000 Grays = 1 kiloGray (1kGy). One kiloGray increases the shelf life of some fruits and vegetables by changing the chemistry of their cells to retard ripening and rotting. Higher doses, 4.75 to 8 kiloGrays, kill salmonella. Very high doses, up to the 30 kGy used to irradiate herbs and spices, render foods sterile.

Food irradiation in the United States was developed primarily at government expense. It started with post–World War II research by the United States army to create good-tasting, economical, shelf-stable field rations for the troops. Interest in food irradiation research and development further expanded in both the government and private sectors during the early to mid 1950s.

Progress slowed somewhat after the passage of the Food Additives Amendment to the Federal Food, Drugs, and Cosmetic Act in 1958. In the amendment, Congress and administrative agencies classified irradiation as a food additive rather than a process since its use affects the characteristics of foods. Therefore, companies wishing to use irradiation were required to petition the FDA for approval. The new use of radiation had to be proven safe with appropriate toxicological studies.

The first approved uses of irradiation occurred in 1963 to preserve canned bacon and to kill insects in wheat and wheat products. In 1964 irradiation of potatoes was allowed to retard sprouting. However, bacon regulations were revoked in 1968 when further evaluation of the data raised doubts that the safety of radiation-sterilized bacon had been demonstrated.

The FDA established the Bureau of Foods Irradiated Food Committee in 1979 to review the agency's policies regarding irradiation and to recommend how to test more accurately for the effects of food irradiation. The committee estimated that a 1 kGy irradiation dose would form "radiolytic products," a class of molecules formed when the ions produced by radiation react with other molecules in the food. Ten percent of these molecules would be unknown compounds. Despite the fact that it takes only one mutant molecule to start a cancer, the committee concluded that at doses below 1kGy, any single "unique" radiolytic product of unusual toxicity would be negligible.

Because it is impossible to test food for the amount of radiation administered, the committee conceded to base their evaluation of irradiation primarily on theoretical estimates extrapolated from radiation chemistry. In 1981 the FDA completely reversed its testing policy, concluding that an adequate margin of safety had been demonstrated for foods irradiated below 1 kGy. Consequently, without the burden of testing, new uses of food irradiation are approved more quickly. To date, approval has been given to irradiate pork, fresh fruits and vegetables, dry or dehydrated enzyme preparations, herbs and spices, and most recently, poultry.

Continuing high-profile food poisoning incidents have begun to interest food processors in using electron and gamma-ray sterilization technologies. The present method of choice uses radioactive isotopes but high-power electron particle accelerators are proving an increasingly attractive alternative. A family of compact industrial continuous-wave linear accelerators are under development which produce electrons with increased energy capacity (Alimov, Knapp, Shvedunov, & Trower, 2000).

Scientific study on irradiation continues. There have been several recent outbreaks of salmonellosis and infections with *Escherichia coli* O157:H7 linked to the consumption of raw sprouts. Ionizing radiation is a process that can be used to reduce the population of pathogens on sprouts. One study investigated ionizing radiation as a means to reduce or to totally inactivate these pathogens, if present, on sprouts. Before inoculation, the sprouts were irradiated to 6 kGy to remove the background microflora. The sprouts were inoculated either with *Salmonella spp.* or with *E. coli* O157:H7. Salmonella was not detected by enrichment culture on sprouts grown from alfalfa seeds naturally contaminated with salmonella after the sprouts were irradiated to a dose of 0.5 kGy or greater (Rajkowski & Thayer, 2000).

ARTIFICIAL SWEETENERS

Artificial sweeteners such as saccharin, cyclamates, and aspartame were developed to replace naturally occurring sugars in food products. In 1981 the FDA banned cyclamates and enforced controls on the use of saccharin. It approved the sale of aspartame, a product 200 times as sweet as sucrose. The most recent product is Splenda (sucrose), a tiny serving of which has zero calories and yields as much sweetness as 2 teaspoons of sugar. In actuality, Splenda is not an artificial sweetener because it is made from a sugar molecule, but it has been chemically changed so the body will not absorb it.

Aspartame is formed by joining two amino acids that are naturally produced by the bacterial breakdown of organic substances. Aspartame has a brief and controversial past. It was accidentally discovered in 1965 when the substance was being studied as a potential ulcer treatment. The USFDA rescinded its original 1974 approval following controversial reports that aspartame, when used to combat obesity, caused brain lesions in laboratory animals. In light of controversies over other artificial sweeteners, chiefly cyclamates and saccharin, the FDA conducted several more years of extensive tests. Aspartame was granted limited approval in 1981 and final approval in 1983. It quickly became an ingredient in many diet foods, especially soft drinks. It is now one of the most frequently used sweeteners in the marketplace.

As you can see, any of these artificial sweeteners can cause problems. However, it is theorized that more people in the United States currently die of obesity-related diseases than of ones related to artificial sweeteners. It is best to limit both your sugar and artificial sweetener consumption, not to choose one over the other.

OLESTRA

Specially manufactured low-fat and nonfat foods have become increasingly available over the past 2 decades and controversy has surrounded the issue of whether these products have beneficial or adverse effects on the health and nutritional status of Americans. One of the best known of these new hybrid products is olestra. Olestra is known as a fat replacer because it is used to replace fat in preparing foods. What makes olestra different is that it is the first nonfat cooking oil or spread with similar properties to fat. Also it does not have to be part of any system to work; it does what it is supposed to do by itself. Like ordinary fat, olestra does not break down when subjected to high temperatures. That means it can be used in cooking and frying, but unlike ordinary fat, olestra is not absorbed when eaten. Instead, it travels through the body unchanged, like any poorly absorbed food components, such as high-fiber bran. One study examined the association of olestra consumption with changes in dietary intakes of energy, fat, and cholesterol and changes in weight and serum lipid concentrations. Data was obtained from 335 participants in the Olestra Post-Marketing Surveillance Study in Marion County (Indianapolis, Indiana). Diet, weight, and serum lipid levels were assessed before the market release of olestra and 1 year later, after olestra-containing foods were widely available. Olestra intake at the 1-year follow-up was categorized as none, low, moderate, and heavy. It was found that participants in the heavy olestra consumption category significantly reduced dietary intake of percentage of energy from fat and saturated fat. Consumers in the highest category of olestra consumption had significantly reduced total serum cholesterol levels compared with olestra nonconsumers. These results indicate that introduction of this new fat substitute in the U.S. market was associated with healthful changes in dietary fat intake and serum cholesterol concentrations among consumers who chose to consume olestra-containing foods (Patterson et al., 2000).

GENETICALLY MODIFIED FOODS

Genetic engineering in agriculture involves splicing a gene from one organism, such as a bacterium, into a plant or animal to confer certain traits, such as drought tolerance or insect resistance in the case of plants. Genetically engineered varieties of soybeans and corn became popular with farmers in the late 1990s and are found in products throughout supermarkets. New herbicide-resistant wheat is due to come on the market in 2003. Biotech varieties of fruit, vegetables, fish, and livestock are in various stages of development.

Under a policy developed during the early 1990s, the FDA considers gene-altered crops to be essentially the same as those produced by conventional breeding methods and thus not subject to the same regulatory controls as food additives. A federal judge upheld the policy in 2000.

In early 2001 the FDA proposed rules that would require biotechnology companies to consult with the government before selling new genetically engineered foods or ingredients. Currently, companies are not required to have the FDA review new biotech crops, although most do so voluntarily. The FDA also proposed voluntary guidelines for food companies to follow if they label foods as biotech-free or promote biotech ingredients. Companies will have to notify FDA of new biotech products at least 4 months before they are to be put on the market.

Scientific descriptions of the new products, including information about genetic modification and the potential to cause allergic reactions, would be posted on the Internet during the agency's review. Some of the data could be kept confidential if companies show FDA the information involves trade secrets. These new rules are in line with a series of proposals made in 2000 to respond to criticism of regulation of the biotech industry. Consumer advocates and environmentalists say federal regulation of the industry is lax and have called for mandatory labeling of all biotech foods.

Biotech and food companies, hoping to head off more stringent regulation, had asked for the new review policy and labeling guidelines. The companies say further regulation is unnecessary and are concerned that mandatory labeling of gene-altered products could raise unnecessary public fears about the foods and strangle the industry. The industry became defensive in 2000 because of nationwide recalls of taco shells that were found to contain a variety of gene-altered corn that had not been approved for human consumption. There remain unresolved questions about whether the StarLink corn could cause allergic reactions. It is the only biotech crop not allowed in food (Lomax, 2000).

The Need for Genetically Modified Foods

Genetically modified (GM) crops offer benefits by reducing waste and agrochemical use in agriculture, and offer the potential of the technology for further crop improvement in the future (Halford & Shewry, 2000). Food production per head in the world as a whole has begun to level off in the last decade, while the world population continues to grow, risking malnutrition, perhaps even starvation, civil unrest, and environmental damage. Very little more land suitable for agriculture is available, and the factors behind the green revolution may not produce further increases. GM crops offer the possibility of increased yields, but also present major problems. In developing countries, where yields are well below what is theoretically possible, the best approach may be better management by small farmers through improvements in their traditional methods. Much more financial support for and research in agriculture is needed, together with more equitable distribution of existing production (Waterlow, 2000).

Why the Concern?

Some of the major concerns of the general public regarding GM crops and food concern: (1) segregation of GM and non-GM crops and cross-pollination between GM crops and wild species; (2) the use of antibiotic resistance marker genes; (3) the possibilities of new allergens being introduced into the food chain; and (4) the relative safety of GM and non-GM foods (Halford & Shewry, 2000).

One usually thinks of plant biology as a noncontroversial topic, but the concerns raised over the biosafety of GM plants have reached disproportionate levels relative to the actual risks. While the technology of changing the genome of plants has been gradually refined and increasingly implemented, the commercialization of GM crops has exploded. Today's commercialized transgenic plants have been produced using *Agrobacterium tumefaciens*-mediated transformation or gene gun-mediated transformation. Recently, incremental improvements of biotechnologies, such as the use of green fluorescent protein (GFP) as a selectable marker, have been developed. Nontransformation genetic modification technologies such as chimeraplasty will be increasingly used to more precisely modify germ plasm. In spite of the increasing knowledge about genetic modification of plants, concerns over ecological and food biosafety have escalated beyond scientific rationality. While several risks associated with GM crops and foods have been identified, the popular press, spurred by colorful protest groups, has left the general public with a sense of imminent danger. Ecological biosafety research has identified potential risks associated with certain crop/transgene combinations, such as intra- and interspecific transgene flow, persistence, and the consequences of transgenes in unintended hosts. Resistance management strategies for insect resistance transgenes and nontarget effects of these genes have also been studied. Food biosafety research has focused on transgenic product toxicity and allergenicity. However, an estimated $3.5 \times 10(12)$ transgenic plants have been grown in the United States in the past 12 years, with over 2 trillion being grown in 1999 and 2000 alone. These large numbers and the absence of any negative reports of compromised biosafety indicate that genetic modification by biotechnology poses no immediate or significant risks and that resulting food products from GM crops are as safe as foods from conventional varieties (Stewart, Richards, & Halfhill, 2000).

Still there is potential for danger. The possible transfer of antibiotic resistance genes from GM plant material to microbes through genetic recombination in the human or animal gut is a consideration that has engendered caution in the use of GM foods (Chiter, Forbes, & Blair, 2000). There also is concern about the safety of GM foods worldwide. One country has suggested that all GM foods should be subjected to long-term animal feeding studies before approval for human consumption (Domingo Roig, & Gomez Arnaiz, 2000).

Social theories of risk suggest that a combination of scientific and cultural perspectives converge to influence risk perception. Some suggest a procedural ethic for public discourse and decision making over the diffusion of GM foods. Ethical and social theories are linked with the hope that by recognizing the social dimensions of debates over new technologies a broader framework for conducting risk analysis may emerge (Lomax, 2000).

Ensuring Safety

It is important to realize that there are legal requirements for containment of novel GM crops and regulatory bodies ensure that GM crops and food are safe (Halford & Shewry, 2000). In addition, scientists know that they have an ongoing duty to conduct objective research and to effectively communicate the results, especially those pertaining to the relative risks and potential benefits, to scientists first and then to the public (Martens, 2000). Finally, health ethicists are dialoguing about both sides of the issue to help determine what is best for people. All stakeholders in the technology will want to maintain open and effective dialogues to better understand risks and benefits of adopting or not adopting agricultural biotechnologies. Health care providers may provide the bridge between the scientists and the consumer in these important nutritional controversies.

SUMMARY

Controversy abounds in a world of change. It is part of the nature of change. In the 21st century, science and technology are evolving more rapidly than ever in the journey of human evolution. Nutrition and what and how we feed a growing world population are at the heart of change, and thus controversy.

When controversy stirs, remember that most fruitful discoveries that have advanced our civilization have occurred in the midst of controversy. However, despite the seal of approval bestowed on controversial products, issues, or foods, it is probably best to use these and other artificial substances in moderate to small amounts.

REFERENCES

Alimov, A. S., Knapp, E. A., Shvedunov, V. I., & Trower, W. P. (2000). High-power CW LINAC for food irradiation. *Applied Radiation and Isotopes, 53*(4–5), 815–820.

Buemann, B., Toubro, S., Raben, A., Blundell, J., & Astrup, A. (2000). The acute effect of D-tagatose on food intake in human subjects. *British Journal of Nutrition, 84*(2), 227–231.

Chiter, A., Forbes, J. M., & Blair, G. E. (2000). DNA stability in plant tissues: Implications for the possible transfer of genes from genetically modified food. *FEBS Letters, 481*(2), 164–168.

Domingo Roig, J. L., & Gomez Arnaiz, M. (2000). Health risks of genetically modified foods: A literature review. *Rev Esp Salud Publication, 74*(3), 255–261.

Halford, N. G., & Shewry, P. R. (2000). Genetically modified crops: Methodology, benefits, regulation and public concerns. *British Medical Bulletin, 56*(1), 62–73.

Lawrence, M., & Rayner, M. (1998). Functional foods and health claims: A public health policy perspective. *Public Health Nutrition, 1*(2), 75–82.

Lomax, G. P. (2000). From breeder reactors to butterflies: Risk, culture, and biotechnology. *Risk Analysis, 20*(5), 747–753.

Martens, M. A. (2000). Safety evaluation of genetically modified foods. *International Archives of Occupational and Environmental Health,73* (Suppl.), S14–18.

O'Brien, M. (2000). Have lessons been learned from the UK bovine spongiform encephalopathy (BSE) epidemic? *International Journal of Epidemiology, 29*(4), 730–733.

Patterson, R. E., Kristal, A. R., Peters, J. C., Neuhouser, M. L., Rock, C. L., Cheskin, L. J., Neumark-Sztainer, D., & Thornquist, M. D. (2000). Changes in diet, weight, and serum lipid levels associated with olestra consumption. *Archives of Internal Medicine, 160*(17), 2600–2604.

Rajkowski, K. T., & Thayer, D. W. (2000). Reduction of *Salmonella spp.* and strains of Escherichia coli O157:H7 by gamma radiation of inoculated sprouts. *Journal of Food Protection, 63*(7), 871–875.

Shea, K. M. (2000). Technical report: Irradiation of food. *Pediatrics, 106*(6), 1505–1510.

Stewart, C. N. Jr., Richards, H. A. 4th, & Halfhill, M. D.(2000). Transgenic plants and biosafety: Science, misconceptions, and public perceptions. *Biotechniques, 29*(4), 832–836, 838–843.

Vaughan, K., & McConaghy, N. (1999). Megavitamin and dietary treatment in schizophrenia: A randomised, controlled trial. *Austalian and New Zealand Journal of Psychiatry, 33*(1), 84–88.

Waterlow, J. (2000). Feeding the world in the new millennium. *Medicine, Conflict, and Survival, 16*(1), 104–107.

Gaining Control of Your Weight

CHAPTER 18

Effective Dieting

Do diets really work? This may be the most perplexing question of the decade. There are literally hundreds of diet plans and countless thousands of people who are on "diets" at this very moment. The unfortunate fact is that 95 percent of them will regain all their lost weight, with proportionately more fat than muscle.

What keeps dieters ready and willing to spend their time, money, and energy on yet another diet is the addictive short-term, rapid weight loss that is possible with virtually every diet on the market. For an idea of the breadth and range of popular diet books, go to any bookstore and look at the titles. At one store I visited recently, there must have been 30 titles devoted to diets alone.

Why do we need diets? Because for the most part U.S. citizens are overweight.

OBESITY

Obesity is now well recognized as a disease in its own right, one which is largely preventable through changes in lifestyle, especially diet. Obesity is a major determinant of many noncommunicable diseases and induces diabetes mellitus (Type 2: non–insulin-dependent), coronary heart disease, and stroke. It increases the risk of several types of cancer, gallbladder disease, musculoskeletal disorders, and respiratory problems. Because these complications are particularly common in those with high abdominal circumference, this measure should be used as an additional indicator for identifying NCD risk.

The World Health Organization has established an international standard for measuring overweight and obesity—the Body Mass Index (BMI), defined as weight (in kg) divided by the square of one's height (in m): kg/m2. For assessing obesity in adult populations, the BMI categories are:

- BMI 25 kg/m2 for overweight (pre-obese: BMI 25–29.9 kg/m2).
- BMI 30 kg/m2 for obesity:
    Class I obese: BMI 30–34.9 kg/m2.
    Class II obese: BMI 35–39.9 kg/m2.
    Class III obese: BMI 40 kg/m2.

Recent media reports state that over half of all Americans are obese. Respected scientific journals validate that there is an epidemic of obesity in the United States (Mokdad et al., 2000), and link chronic diseases to the problem (Vgontzas, Bixler, Papanicolaou, & Chrousos, 2000). There are clinical differences between lean and obese patients (Weber, Neutel, & Smith, 2001). Obesity has serious health and economic consequences, and finding ways to combat it deserves the attention of all health care professionals.

The Lifetime Health and Economic Consequences of Obesity

The lifetime health and economic consequences of obesity for individual patients has recently been documented (Thompson, Edelsberg, Colditz, Bird, & Oster, 1999). This study tested the relationship between body mass index and the risks and associated costs of five obesity-related diseases: hypertension, hypercholesterolemia, Type II diabetes mellitus, coronary heart disease (CHD), and stroke. Using data from the Third National Health and Nutrition Examination Survey, the Framingham Heart Study, and other secondary sources, the study model estimated:

1. risks of hypertension, hypercholesterolemia, and Type II diabetes mellitus at future ages.
2. lifetime risks of CHD and stroke.
3. life expectancy.
4. expected lifetime medical care costs of these five diseases for men and women age 35 to 64 years with body mass indexes of nonobese and mildly, moderately, and severely obese, respectively.

The findings were that disease risks and costs increase substantially with increased body mass index. The risk of hypertension for moderately obese 45- to 54-year-old men, for example, is roughly two-fold higher than for their nonobese peers, whereas the risk of Type II diabetes mellitus is almost three-fold higher. Lifetime risks of CHD and stroke are similarly elevated, whereas life expectancy is reduced by 1 year. Total discounted lifetime medical care costs for the treatment of these five diseases are estimated to differ by $10,000 ($29,600 versus $19,600). Similar results were obtained for women. The conclusion of this study is that the lifetime health and economic consequences of obesity are substantial and suggest that efforts to prevent or reduce this problem might yield significant benefits (Thompson et al., 1999).

Food Craving and Food Addiction

Although certain commonalties exist between eating and drug use (mood effects, external cue-control of appetites, reinforcement, and so on), it is argued that the vast majority of cases of self-reported food craving and food "addiction" should not be viewed as addictive behavior. An explanation is proposed that instead gives a prominent role to the psychological processes of ambivalence and attribution, operating together with normal mechanisms of appetite control, the hedonic effects of certain foods, and socially and culturally determined perceptions of appropriate intakes and uses of those foods. Ambivalence about foods such as chocolate arises from the attitude that it is highly palatable but should be eaten with restraint. Attempts to restrict intake, however, cause the desire for chocolate to become more salient, an experience that is then labeled as a craving. This, together with a need to provide a reason for why resisting eating chocolate is difficult and sometimes fails, can in turn lead the individual to an explanation in terms of addiction (e.g., "chocoholism"). Moreishness ("causing a desire for more") occurs during rather than preceding an eating episode, and is experienced when the eater attempts to limit consumption before appetite for the food has been sated (Rogers & Smit, 2000).

Dietary Treatments of Obesity

Numerous dietary treatments that purport to offer something unique for stimulating weight loss have been published. These treatments include fad diets, diets formulated by various commercial slimming clubs, very-low-carbohydrate diets (VLCD) and conventional diets. Fad diets may possibly reduce some weight short-term; however, there is no scientific basis to their long-term effectiveness. Commercial slimming clubs may be suitable for some individuals but they need to be properly assessed professionally. There are specific guidelines for the use of VLCD, which are only appropriate for short-term use. There is scientific evidence to suggest that conventional diets can produce both short- and long-term weight loss. A successful weight-loss program depends on a multidisciplinary team approach. Management strategies should be devised for addressing issues such as goals, monitoring, follow-up, relapse, and evaluation. Initial assessments should include medical, laboratory data, fitness level, and dietary and behavioral attitudes. These data will form the basis of the treatment plan. Frequent visits to the clinic are fundamental in promoting continuing weight loss during the long-term maintenance stage of treatment. The visits should be made worthwhile for the patient. Realistic and attainable goals for diet, exercise, and behavior modification should be made. The diet should have a novel approach and be tailored to the needs of the patient. It should be adequate nutritionally, low in carbohydrates and fat. The overall aim should be to promote lifelong changes in lifestyle, improvement in quality of life, and reduction of health risks (Moloney, 2000).

Obesity is a chronic disease, and in most cases weight reduction is the first treatment for its concomitant conditions of hyperlipidemia, diabetes, and hypertension. Weight-reduction diets are controversial in both the popular press and among clinicians treating hyperlipidemia and obesity. Both high-carbohydrate/low-fat and higher-protein/low-carbohydrate diets will produce loss of body fat if the calorie level is low enough. But selecting effective diet prescriptions for bariatric patients requires understanding of both the science and art of nutrition. Low-calorie diets, protein-sparing modified fasts, and modified-carbohydrate diets seem to be the most effective for patient compliance, and modified-carbohydrate plans are probably necessary for maintenance of the weight loss (Holtmeier & Seim, 2000).

Some weight-loss diets are nutritionally sound and consistent with recommendations for healthy eating while others are fad diets encouraging irrational and, sometimes, unsafe practices.

HOW FAD DIETS WORK

During the first few days of a severely reduced-calorie diet, weight seemingly drops off at a substantially satisfying rate. But instead of losing fat, our bodies are consuming their temporary energy reserve (glycogen), which weighs about a pound, and when associated water, weighs another 3 to 4 pounds. The temporary diet is over when our hunger returns and the glycogen is restored as soon as we consume food. Our bodies then readjust for the water deficit, and we regain the weight just as quickly as it was lost.

Any diet that promises a weight loss of more than 1 to 2 pounds per week is either counting on this very temporary rapid weight loss or on a prolonged diet plan that restricts calories below 1,200, the minimum amount we need for basic metabolic processes. While it is possible to increase metabolism to help whittle away stored fat calories, severely restricting intake is not the way to do it.

One of the primary determinants of the body's basal metabolic rate is the proportion of lean muscle to fat tissue. Each pound of muscle burns 30 to 50 calories a day to stay alive, while fat burns only 2 calories per pound a day. When a diet offers too few calories to support basal metabolic rate, our bodies choose to hold on to precious fat molecules for what they perceive to be famine times ahead and switch to lean muscle tissue for fuel. Consequently, our metabolic rate slackens to conserve energy for this new survival mode. Restricted food intake also supplies inadequate nutrients for optimum health and energy.

POPULAR DIET PLANS

It is not within the scope or intent of this book to elaborate on specific diets, but it is important to realize that thousands, perhaps millions of people, currently follow one or more of the well-known diet plans. You probably have heard of some of them or maybe even tried one or more of them yourself. Pritikin, Weight Watchers, Jenny Craig, and the grapefruit diet plan are examples of but a few. Some of these popular commercial diet programs do work toward whole body health by advocating exercise and/or stress management programs along with their eating plan. Some of the more intriguing programs and their lively leaders, such as Susan Powter, advocate complete lifestyle change to remake ourselves. The point to remember here is that some of these diets do work for some people. Not all of us are alike, however, so many of us need to look in alternative directions.

Comparison of Eight Popular Diets and Their Potential Long-Term Weight Loss

One study compared several weight-loss diets and assessed their potential long-term effects. Eight popular weight-loss diets were selected and clinically analyzed to predict their relative benefits/potential harm; these diets were: Atkins, Protein Power, Sugar Busters, Zone, ADA Exchange, High-Fiber Fitness, Pritikin, and Ornish. A summary description, menu plan, and recommended snacks were developed for each diet. The nutrient composition of each diet was determined using computer software, and a Food Pyramid Score was calculated to compare diets. The Mensink, Hegsted, and other formulae were applied to estimate coronary heart disease risk factors. The findings were that higher fat diets are higher in saturated fats and cholesterol than current dietary guidelines and their long-term use will increase serum cholesterol levels and risk for CHD. Diets restricted in sugar intake lower serum cholesterol levels and long-term risk for CHD; however, higher carbohydrate, higher fiber, lower fat diets have the greatest effect in decreasing serum cholesterol concentrations and risk of CHD. While high fat diets may promote short-term weight loss, the potential hazards for worsening risk for progression of atherosclerosis override the short-term benefits. Individuals derive the greatest health benefits from diets low in saturated fat and high in carbohydrate and fiber; these increase sensitivity to insulin and lower risk for CHD (Anderson, Konz, & Jenkins, 2000).

The American Institute for Cancer Research Fad Diet Evaluations

The American Institute for Cancer Research (AICR) evaluated four of the most popular diets as propagated in the authors' diet books. AICR analyzed the potential effectiveness and possible health risks associated with each plan and discovered that all four share many of the same basic characteristics, and that is that they all illustrate the limitations of fad diets in general. The four diets were:

- *Dr. Atkins New Diet Revolution,* by Dr. Robert Atkins.
- *The New Beverly Hills Diet,* by Judy Mazel and Michael Wyatt.
- *Protein Power,* by Michael Eades, MD, and Mary Anne Eades, MD.
- *Suzanne Somers' Get Skinny on Fabulous Food,* by Suzanne Somers.

COMMON DENOMINATORS

All four of the plans reviewed are essentially low calorie diets. None are advertised as such, however. In fact, each encourages the dieter to eat as much as he or she wants of a particular food. Nevertheless, these diets prescribe a daily caloric intake that is well below average requirements. By omitting certain foods, and sometimes even entire food groups, these diets are deficient in such major nutrients as dietary fiber and carbohydrates, as well as in selected vitamins, minerals, and protective phytochemicals. Dr. Atkins, for one, recommends supplementing the diet with nutritional supplements—and helpfully offers his own line of products.

The diets are also out of balance, prescribing a daily dietary intake that is high in protein and fat and low in carbohydrates. These proportions are a far cry from those recommended by AICR and other major health organizations such as the American Heart Association and the American Dietetic Association, as well as the Surgeon General and the U.S. Department of Agriculture (USDA). On a practical level, such high-protein, high-fat, low-carbohydrate diets tend to promote the loss of water weight. However much this diuretic effect may engender a false sense of accomplishment in the dieter, this weight can and does return quickly.

If such an imbalanced diet is maintained, the body soon reverts to a fasting state called ketosis, in which the body begins to metabolize muscle tissue instead of fat. Authors of these diets actually advocate "taking advantage" of ketosis to hasten weight loss. In fact, this state is one of the body's last-ditch emergency responses; deliberately inducing ketosis can lead to muscle breakdown, nausea, dehydration, headaches, light-headedness, irritability, bad breath, and kidney problems. In pregnancy, ketosis may cause fetal abnormality or death. It can be fatal in individuals who have diabetes.

Over an extended period of time, all four diets can give rise to other health risks, as well. By restricting carbohydrates, all four diets inevitably lead to a lack of fiber, which can cause constipation and other gastrointestinal difficulties. In addition, the high amounts of cholesterol and saturated fat they prescribe increase the risk of heart disease and, possibly, some cancers. There is recent evidence that a diet featuring excessive protein may leach calcium from the bones. Over and above these health risks, however, two of the diets discussed in Table 18–1 promote baseless ideas about food combinations. The elaborate case they make for eating specific foods in a specific order and at specific times has no nutritional basis, and amounts to a kind of magical thinking.

WHY FAD DIETS DO NOT WORK

The notion of the quick fix is central to all fad diets. So, too, is the mistaken belief that a change in our bodies can result only from a radical change in how we eat. Most people look to these diet plans not for help making gradual, long-term adjustments to overall lifestyle, but to loose excess weight in about 2 weeks.

PERMANENT WEIGHT LOSS

If you are serious about permanent weight loss and weight maintenance, you do not want a quick-fix, weight reduction plan. Instead you must employ all your body-mind-spirit resources to change or modify your lifestyle. Weight loss without long-term behavior change will fail. The weight will return and the roller coaster process will begin anew. A diet plan that includes exercise, a change in attitudes, and an alteration in causative behaviors is the only thing that will work for the long term. Implementing a plan of healing nutrition into a healthy life plan can bring about miraculous whole body changes.

Some people find that the Dean Ornish diet for a healthy heart works for them. Basically a macrobiotic (meatless) diet, Ornish teaches converts to eliminate meat, fat, and most sugars while incorporating an exercise and stress management plan. Other nutritionists such as Jeffrey Bland and Jonathan Wright have developed their own specialty diet regimens. Each of these plans works for some people, especially the ones who are serious about weight management.

The word *diet* originally comes from the Greek *diaita,* which means "manner of living." Scientists and nutritionists agree that any long-term program of weight loss and maintenance must be more than a matter of rationing carbohydrates and calculating calories. It must extend to the entire lifestyle plan.

The AICR recommendations, called the Diet and Health Guidelines for Cancer Prevention, include eight steps:

1. Choose a diet rich in a variety of plant-based foods.
2. Eat plenty of vegetables and fruits.
3. Maintain a healthy weight and be physically active.
4. Drink alcohol in moderation, if at all.

TABLE 18–1 Evaluation of Four Fad Diets*

DR. ATKINS' NEW DIET REVOLUTION

This diet is an update of Dr. Atkins' previous diet, recycled here perhaps to encourage the sale of dietary supplements. Besides the health risks associated with ketosis outlined earlier, there are other long-term concerns associated with this particular plan.

Atkins' diet can lead to the kind of rapid weight fluctuations that adversely affect the heart. Moreover, the breakdown of fatty acids that occurs during ketosis may also increase the risk of heart disease.

One of the basic tenets of Atkins' diet is that sugar causes cancer. Such misleading pronouncements are essentially scare tactics, meant to direct the dieter towards foods on the Atkins plan.

Finally, nothing about this plan encourages the dieter to learn some very basic weight management strategies like portion control and serving sizes, let alone develop the skills necessary for a lifetime of balanced nutrition.

THE NEW BEVERLY HILLS DIET

Ms. Mazel, the diet's author, has no health or nutrition credentials. Her New Beverly Hills Diet is fundamentally flawed, which curtails any potential long-term effectiveness and even gives rise to certain risks. Specifically, two of Ms. Mazel's theories about digestion are wrong.

The premise of her diet is that enzymes found in food "activate" the human body. Each of the three food groups—proteins, carbohydrates, and fats—contain their own set of enzymes to break down food so that the body can properly digest it.

Her diet advocates a practice termed *Cautious Combining*. "It is when you eat and what foods you eat together that matters." Fruits, for example, contain all of the enzymes necessary to break themselves down into nutrients, and move quickly through the system. Proteins and carbohydrates, however, require special enzymes that slow down the process.

Furthermore, enzymes from one food can't "cross over" to work on other food groups. These suppositions are incorrect. The enzymes necessary for digestion are found within the body, not in the foods we eat.

Her diet also states that fat is just another symptom of indigestion, that when food is not properly digested, it "causes fatness." In fact, quite the opposite is true—if foods are not properly digested they cannot be absorbed. If they are not absorbed, they cannot be metabolized—into fat or anything else.

PROTEIN POWER

Protein Power gets the most credit for providing sound starting points for weight loss. The authors advise getting a physical exam, setting realistic base

*Adapted from material from the American Institute for Cancer Research. Web address: http//www.airc.org. Reprinted with permission.

TABLE 18–1	**Evaluation of Four Fad Diets** *(continued)*

lines involving body fat percentages and ideal body weight, relying on internal perceptions rather than the bathroom scale, keeping a food diary, and drinking lots of water. The diet itself, however, places the individual at risk for many of the same problems seen in the other diets examined.

The plan's directive to consume 25 grams of fiber daily while maintaining a low-carbohydrate intake is effectively impossible, as most high fiber foods contain significant amounts of carbohydrates.

The name of the plan itself, Protein Power, is misleading. The authors recommend 60 grams of protein a day for a relatively active individual with a lean body mass of 100 pounds. But 60 grams of protein is nothing more than the USDA recommended daily allowance for a person of that weight. In fact, the average American normally eats around 100 grams of protein a day. The Protein Power plan simply cuts carbohydrates, producing what is essentially a low-calorie diet.

The authors blame insulin for a host of ills, including hypertension, heart disease, elevated cholesterol, and diabetes. High insulin levels, they say, lead to weight gain and obesity. In fact, the scientific evidence suggests that being obese causes high insulin levels, not the other way around.

SUSANNE SOMERS' GET SKINNY ON FABULOUS FOOD

Before she began penning diet books, the only remotely health-related entry on Suzanne Somers' résumé was an infomercial for a thigh exerciser. She brings no nutrition credentials to bear on this book, which blames excess fat on the tendency of the body's enzymes to "cancel each other out." Her solution, a Byzantine process of eliminating "Funky Foods" and separating the rest into "Somersized Food Groups" for mixing and matching, has no nutritional basis.

Somers maintains that when proteins and carbohydrates are eaten together, their enzymes "cancel each other out," creating a halt in the digestion process and causing weight gain. Unfortunately, this reasoning is based on assumptions that are completely false. In fact, the body contains enzymes that are specifically keyed to individual proteins, carbohydrates, and fats. These enzymes do not "cancel each other out," because they remain in different areas of the digestive tract.

If digestion did not occur, the resulting lack of protein and carbohydrate absorption would most likely result in weight loss, not the weight gain Somers' predicts. Somers' advice not to drink water with meals because it dilutes the digestive juices and slows digestion is also without merit.

In most other particulars, the Somers' plan closely resembles the other three diets, and places the dieter at similar risk.

5. Select foods low in fat and salt.

6. Prepare and store foods safely.

7. Do not smoke or use tobacco in any form.

8. Engage in regular physical exercise.

Portion Control and Serving Sizes

Portion size is a concept that most fad diets do not address. Many call for the elimination of whole categories of macronutrients but ignore this basic nutritional concept. In fact, to lose weight without jeopardizing health, most people should maintain the standard proportion of macronutrients (more carbohydrates from plant-based foods, less protein and fat from animal-based foods.) At the same time, they should increase daily exercise levels and decrease portion sizes.

In general, all Americans need to be aware of portion size, even those not expressly looking to lose weight. Researchers say that Americans routinely underestimate how many calories they consume each day by as much as 25 percent. Busy lifestyles mean countless distractions. Many of us eat on the run, at our desks, or in front of the television. Individual portions are difficult to gauge when our attention is divided.

In addition, fast-food chains compete for our business by inflating their serving sizes. Modestly sized bagels and muffins have all but disappeared from American cafés, replaced by creations three or four times larger. Restaurants are not far behind, using larger plates laden with more food to assure customers they're getting their money's worth. Of course, these trends are merely symptoms; how much food we eat is ultimately up to us. We've simply forgotten when to say when, and so lost sight of a fundamental concept of everyday nutrition: the serving size.

Portion size is on the label of every food package. It is the basic unit of measure used by dietitians and health organizations across the United States. It lies at the center of every discussion of balanced diets and weight management, but few of us know how much food a "serving size" represents. To put serving sizes in perspective, see the list of examples that follows. Serving sizes are much smaller than most Americans realize. According to the USDA, one serving equals:

- 1 slice of whole-grain bread
- ½ cup of cooked rice or pasta
- 3–4 small crackers
- 1 small pancake or waffle
- 2 medium-sized cookies
- ½ cup cooked or raw vegetables
- 1 cup (4 leaves) lettuce
- 1 small baked potato

- ¾ cup vegetable juice
- 1 medium apple
- ½ grapefruit or mango
- ½ cup berries
- 1 cup yogurt or milk
- 1½ ounces of cheddar cheese
- 1 chicken breast
- 1 medium pork chop
- ¼ pound hamburger patty

The USDA list, helpful as it is, is only one way to get a handle on portions. In 1993 the USDA redesigned food labels to make it easier to gauge serving sizes—and thus calories, fat, protein, and nutrients. In addition, they mandated that serving sizes be clearly stated and consistent for all foods in a given product line. The redesigned Nutrition Facts labels (see Figure 11–1 on p. 138) appear on most every packaged food product made in the United States.

The USDA lists and food labels are excellent sources of information for proper portion control, but the most important way to manage how much you're taking in is to develop an eye for serving sizes. Gaining the knack is easier than it sounds; it doesn't mean breaking out the measuring cups and spoons every time you prepare a meal or dine out. AICR recommends two quick ways to become conversant with this important nutritional concept.

RULES OF THUMB

The key is to translate the abstract information represented by the serving size into something visual that's easily remembered. So instead of trying to memorize lists of ounce, cup, and tablespoon equivalents, simply relate the serving sizes of various foods to familiar physical objects. Here are some tried-and-true rules of thumb.

THE EYEBALL METHOD

The single best way to determine the amount of food in a given serving is to consult the Nutrition Facts label and measure it out. Of course, measuring every food at each meal is not a particularly practical or enjoyable option, so AICR recommends taking a day to eyeball your servings. Check the label, and fill a measuring cup with the appropriately sized portion of vegetables, or chicken, or rice, or snacks. Then empty it onto a plate, and take a good look. How much of the plate is covered? What, exactly, does one serving of pasta look like? Meat? Sauce? Even if you do this only once, in those few seconds you'll arm yourself with information vital to achieving your weight-management goals. By refocusing attention on an often-overlooked variable in the dieting equation, this method provides a simple and effective reference point. If you've been eating more than you realize, the calories and fat grams steadily add up; sooner or later, the pounds follow. Even if you're not trying to lose weight, taking a moment to see how many servings of cereal you actually eat each morning could help you structure your daily intake.

Once you develop a sense for servings, you'll find controlling your weight and balancing your diet become easier. You might still load up on your favorite foods once in a while, but you'll be fully aware that you are doing so, and that's the key. Paying attention to portions means eliminating the kind of unconscious eating that has helped lead to the current U.S. weight crisis.

Here are some ways to put your newly developed powers of portion control into effect. At home:

- Use smaller dishes at meals.
- Avoid serving food family style. Serve up plates with appropriate portions in the kitchen, and don't go back for seconds.
- Put away any leftovers quickly, in separate, portion-controlled amounts. This makes it harder to sneak extra-large helpings later on.
- Never eat out of the bag or carton.

At restaurants:

- Ask for half or smaller portions. Don't worry if it doesn't seem cost-effective—it's worth it.
- Eyeball your appropriate portion, set the rest aside, and ask for a doggie bag right away. Servings are so big at many restaurants that you may wind up with lunch for two days.
- At buffets, do a little reconnaissance. Walk the length of the buffet table from the desserts to the appetizers to see your options. Select only those foods that truly appeal, and keep the rules of thumb in mind. If, for example, you want to try several different kinds of fish, make sure to keep the amounts small enough so that, together, they still fit inside a checkbook-sized serving.
- If you have dessert, share. (Remember that many restaurant desserts look better than they taste.)

At the supermarket:

- Beware of mini-snacks—tiny crackers, cookies, pretzels. Most people end up eating more than they realize, and the calories add up.
- Choose foods packaged in individual serving sizes. Again, the extra money you spend is worth the calories you are likely to save.
- If you're the type who eats ice cream out of the carton, pick up ice cream sandwiches or other individual size servings.

BREAKING OLD HABITS, SUBSTITUTING NEW BEHAVIORS

Behavioral therapists say that it takes 21 days to develop a new habit. Just as it is easier to sew an entirely new dress than remake an old one, it takes longer to abandon old ingrained, bad habits and rebuild them than it does to begin from scratch. So it is with our eating habits. If, for example, you have been drinking caffeinated soft drinks, eating donuts for mid-morning snacks, and having your main meal in the evening for a decade or more, it may take a while to change this routine.

Willpower

Willpower is one of the most important aspects of dieting. Willpower is what makes diets work and what helps us to achieve what we want. Let us talk about willpower and food and willpower and emotions. What does the word *willpower* really mean? Does it mean that we have to deny ourselves time to relax at the end of the day because we have to jog to keep our bodies exercised to live longer? Does it mean we cannot go to an after-hours party because we promised to take the kids to a ball game? Or does it simply mean determination?

I propose that willpower is what we use to get ahead in life. Willpower is what we use along with determination, whether it be to get our bodies healthy or to make a million dollars. We all know people who constantly complain about their weight, their diets, or their lives. Those of us who have willpower do something about the situation. For example, we might throw out the junk food in our cabinets or go skating or dancing if we are dieting. Willpower is what will change our lives and our eating habits. We have all heard this before, yet it is a true statement. We must have willpower to succeed.

How do we get willpower to diet? First, let's talk of situations. You are sitting at the table tonight and you have made or bought a cake for dessert. Go ahead, have a small piece. When you want another, just say this word loud and clear in your head—*no*! Put the dessert in the freezer or give it away. Go on with life, and within a day you will have forgotten it. At this point, start saying no to other high-fat, high-calorie foods. By doing this, you will begin saying yes to a lot more.

This is the only life you have, unless you believe in reincarnation, and of course, you want to make the best of it. By making yourself what you want to be, you will know and be satisfied that you have accomplished something. Although it may seem strange to find a willpower chapter in a book on nutrition, this book is not just about food, it is about you. You must look at every aspect of yourself to understand the relationship between food and yourself and how to develop the willpower to control it. Try the following steps to boost your willpower:

1. Think about what you really want.
2. Think about why you want it.
3. Realize that willpower is your way to get it, whether it is a lower weight or a healthier body.
4. Do what you know is best, not what your taste buds tell you.

Creative Visualization

A creative way to follow through on willpower is to utilize an imagery or visualization experience before you eat. Try this exercise prior to your next meal.

Take a long, slow, deep breath in through your nose. Hold your breath as you count to four, and then exhale through your mouth. As you follow this breathing pattern one more time, read the following script:

- I am totally and completely relaxed.
- I am losing from 2 to 7 pounds per month. I am losing weight consistently until I reach my goal.
- I am eating less and enjoying it more.
- Both my appetite and hunger are satisfied quickly.
- I am leaving food on my plate and feel good about it.
- I am losing pounds consistently each month until I reach my weight goal.
- I can see myself as I will look when I reach my ideal weight.
- All these suggestions are becoming a part of me and are effective now.

Food Diary

It is often difficult to recall just what you ate and when you ate it. Attempting to recall specific foods at specific times may block your ability to relate eating behaviors to being overweight. Before beginning to diet, as well as once you are underway, you will probably find it helpful to record what you eat. In this way, you will have an hour-by-hour record of what you actually ate, not just what you remember. It is amazing how easily we can forget the actual quantities and types of food we ate just 24 hours ago. A food diary recording is an excellent guide for you as you begin to modify eating behaviors. Table 18–2 depicts a simple recording schedule that you can copy into a notebook. The idea is simply to put in writing everything that you put into your mouth. This is the only way you can really know your actual intake.

Food Cravings

Sometimes despite our best intentions, it seems impossible to apply willpower when we crave high-calorie foods.

TABLE 18–2	Food Diary	

DATE	TIME	FOOD CONSUMED
_____	6:00 A.M.	_____
	7:00	_____
	8:00	_____
	9:00	_____
	10:00	_____
	11:00	_____
	Noon	_____
	1:00 P.M.	_____
	2:00	_____
	3:00	_____
	4:00	_____
	5:00	_____
	6:00	_____
	7:00	_____
	8:00	_____
	9:00	_____
	10:00	_____
	11:00	_____
	Midnight	_____
	1:00 A.M.– 6:00 A.M.	_____

CASE STUDY: Betty

Betty worked nights in the hospital telemetry unit. She had been out of school for 3 years and, much to her chagrin, had gained 60 pounds. When she met with the dietitian for the first time, she did not intend to delve into her nutritional habits. She simply wanted a quick physical assessment and the okay to begin an exercise class. The dietitian strongly

(Continued on next page)

suggested that in addition to the exercise class, Betty return for weekly nutritional counseling sessions.

During the weekly sessions, Betty's eating patterns unfolded. After work at 7:00 A.M., she went home, made breakfast for her family, and got the children off to school. Then she ate the leftovers, cleaned the kitchen, and went to bed. She was up at 4:00 P.M. to greet the kids with an afternoon snack. Later, she made supper and ate a leisurely meal with her family. The dietitian soon discovered that the problem eating time came during the night. By the time Betty arrived at work, she had met all her caloric requirements for the day. Betty and her nurse colleagues had started working the same shift at the same time and had worked together continuously for 3 years. They had acquired the pattern of each one bringing in a covered dish every night so they could eat a communal "supper" at 2:00 A.M. and pastries before the last flurry of activities at 5:00 A.M. They also drank copious quantities of coffee throughout the night. To add spice to their lives, they "dressed up" their coffee with fancy commercial creams. They took turns bringing in the cream. As you might suspect, the dairy creamers got fancier and fancier. At first they used nondairy creamer, then half and half, but a year ago they began using the speciality coffee creamers in the pint-size milk cartons. Amaretto, Irish Cream, and Swiss Mocha flavors were among their favorites. The craving for coffee and creamers became an unconscious addiction. Without thinking, Betty added the creamers to her coffee at home and insisted on real cream in her coffee when she ate out.

It was not until the dietitian explained the high-fat, high-calorie content to Betty that she became aware of how much additional intake she was consuming. Betty reported her insights to her colleagues on the unit and solicited their input for dieting strategies. They too had become fat.

The group devised a plan for cream elimination and gradual coffee withdrawal. Since they realized they had all developed both caffeine and fat addictions, they agreed to tackle the problem together. Over a 3-month period, they substituted skim milk for cream, changed to low-calorie nutritional snacks to replace their 2:00 A.M. supper, and changed from caffeinated coffee to decaffeinated coffee. After 6 months, they had completely revolutionized their nighttime eating habits and had begun to shed pounds. Two of the three nurses also began exercise classes to augment the new lifestyle.

Observation

Cravings usually creep up on us. Our insidious behaviors can develop into food addictions without our realizing what is happening. The following list of activities may help to combat food cravings:

(Continued on next page)

1. *Bring the food craving into conscious awareness.*
2. *Begin a food diary to decipher what events trigger the eating behavior.*
3. *Try to sublimate the desire to eat into another productive behavior. When the desire to eat a high-fat food strikes you, be prepared in advance to substitute another activity or desire. For example, if you have been wanting to take a weekend trip but cannot afford it, start saving money. Each time you want to spend 50 cents on a candy bar or soft drink, put the money in your portable piggy bank instead. You may be surprised at how quickly the funds add up and how soon you will be able to reward yourself because of the substituted behavior.*
4. *Volunteer to work in a soup kitchen or homeless shelter. Spend a shift or two a week serving meals. The psychological impact of this technique has proved beneficial for many who are breaking food craving patterns.*

WHEN AND HOW TO DIET

There are numerous ways to diet. The one you choose will depend on your personality type. In this section, we will see how dieting worked for several different people.

Dieting Alone

A way that works well for some is the isolation method. Those who follow this route virtually retreat from their everyday lives, buy a quantity of diet food, and do not go out.

CASE STUDY: Laura

Laura was an active head nurse on an oncology unit. In addition to her high-pressure job, she was the single parent of two teenage girls. Despite the nagging efforts of her slender daughters, Laura could not summon the willpower to stop eating. At work she was bombarded by the sweets left by well-meaning families and pastries served at staff parties and meetings. In the evenings at home, she was tired and felt she needed a good supper

(Continued on next page)

with her daughters. While trying to relax at night, she was exposed to television advertisements for foods and could not resist snacking and having an occasional mixed drink. After all, she was so tired and food was so comforting. Month after month, despite periodic attempts to diet, her overweight poundage persisted and some months she even gained weight.

One August, in a fury of disgust over what she had become, Laura made a rapid decision. She decided to get away from work, the kids, the house, and the TV and leave town. She recalled her misery following her divorce when the children were young. She remembered how her mother offered to keep the girls so that she could go on a vacation and snap out of her depression. It had worked. She had connected with a local scuba divers club organizing a group trip and had gone to a Mexican island to snorkle. She even had a miserable cold when she departed. The warm January sunshine, the tropical waters, and the group camaraderie had soon broken Laura's cold and the long-standing depression. She had been able to put her life problems into perspective, made new friends, and developed a new skill. By the end of the week, Laura had experienced a miraculous change in her body-mind-spirit health and returned to her home and career responsibilities with a new outlook.

Now, 8 years later, Laura decided she needed another retreat from her immediate environment. This time she was not depressed, she was just fat. She asked one of her friends to look after the girls and arranged for leave from work. Since it was off-season, she was able to get good rates at a seaside resort close to the Mexican border in the same area where she had made a turnaround before. She loaded her car with a stock of good books, motivational tapes, and simple clothes. While driving to the beach, she crunched on carrot and celery sticks and rice cakes and drank one-calorie, caffeine-free, soft drinks.

Once in town, Laura ignored the billboards for fast foods and fancy seafood restaurants and drove directly to the grocery store. She stocked up on low-calorie drinks, fresh fruits and vegetables, fresh eggs, and low-calorie crunchy snacks. She bought no-fat, low-calorie margarine and breads to spread it on. She knew it would take a few days to shrink her massive stomach back to normal size, so she loaded up on foods that would contain bulk but not fats or calories. Armed with bags of diet groceries, Laura retreated to her seaside condominium and began her diet.

She figured that as long as she was retreating to diet she might as well work on her mental and spiritual health at the same time. She began to practice a meditation technique she had learned in college but never seemed to have time for in her busy life. In three days time, Laura read two novels, wrote three letters, swam in the pool, briskly walked the beach twice a day, and began to feel the lethargy ease from her heavy frame.

(Continued on next page)

Television was declared a demon and she consciously unplugged it. She knew that the food ads broke even the most sterling willpower. She was determined not to succumb to the commercials designed to make America fat. She used her free evening time to stroll the beach and sit at the waves' edge to reflect on her past and contemplate her future.

On the fourth day, Laura awoke feeling invigorated. On this day, she developed a long-range planning schedule and then followed her previous days' routine. On the fifth day, she tested herself in the outside world. She drove to a large public cafeteria for her major midday meal. Here she discovered she could buy any combination of four salads or vegetables for a modest price. Since she had declared this retreat week meatless, as well as alcohol-free, this was perfect. She purchased two salads, two hot vegetables, and a tall glass of un-iced water. Positioning herself at a window table, she ate slowly, savoring the hot vegetables. She ate the cold, crisp, carrot and raisin salad for dessert. She boxed the green salad to take home for the evening meal. Laura left the cafeteria full and happy. She had passed the test of the temptation to overindulge.

Laura rounded out the sixth day of her retreat beachcombing, swimming, and enjoying small portions of healthy, nutritious foods. On the seventh day, armed with carrots, celery, rice cakes, and a thermos of water, she drove back home. She felt psychologically stronger, mentally alert, spiritually attuned, and physically ready to begin a long-term eating program that would restore her to a state of vibrant health. She calculated that she spent $500 for the week and considered the cost well worth the self-esteem, self-confidence, and whole body health that she had generated.

Observation

Laura created a situation in which she could isolate herself from responsibilities in the fast-paced world and engage in a 7-day purification, renewal diet. She had the willpower to distance herself from alcohol, caffeine, and high-fat, high-calorie foods and the knowledge to choose what kinds of foods to eat. She created a support system by using motivational audiotapes, withdrawing from television, and including the healing properties of a natural environment. Laura took no scale or measuring tape to monitor her progress because she knew she needed a long-term plan, not short-term calibrations.

For many, separation from the routine daily environment can make a significant difference. Thoughtful isolation can create the space to consider what got you into this condition in the first place and what forces you need in order to move to a more desirable state.

Dieting with a Buddy or Team

Most people are highly social beings and need the support of others to boost their willpower.

CASE STUDY: Sandra

Sandra was an evening staff nurse in the neonatal intensive care unit. She was in her thirties, unmarried, and was, by her own admission, in a rut. Two months ago she had broken off a long-term relationship with her live-in boyfriend. Neither he nor anything else in her life seemed to be on the right track. Since the breakup two months ago, Sandra had moped around with a sense of ennui and fatigue. Her weight problem had not really concerned her until an event in the unit got her attention. Several overweight nurses from all the shifts in her unit decided to hold a contest. By the time the rules were established, 10 nurses agreed to contribute $20 each and see who could lose the most weight in a 3-month period. The winner would collect the $200 prize winnings. Sandra decided to join the pool. Perhaps she could finally concentrate and have a worthy personal goal.

All of the contestants weighed in and had their weight recorded every week. Several of the contestants teamed up together and developed a group strategy and plan. Sandra decided to go the Weight Watchers route. She went to their weekly meetings, bought their food, and became a true convert to their lifestyle change approach to the problem. They suggested she join a local exercise club. This caused her to change her daily schedule. Before she had slept from 2:00 A.M. to 10:00 A.M., had a leisurely breakfast, and watched TV before getting ready for work in the afternoon. After joining the exercise club, she changed her routine and began regular morning workout classes. She made new friends with other Weight Watcher associates and felt as if she was starting her life all over again.

At the end of 3 months, Sandra won the contest. Not only had she lost the most weight in the group of her nursing colleagues, but she had established a network of new health-seeking friends. She collected the $200 prize and took her competitors out for an evening of miniature golf.

Observation

Sandra is typical of many of us. We eat and gain weight often without realizing how or when it happened. She was alert to the situation and

(Continued on next page)

*seized the opportunity to do something about it. We all need social con-
nections and friendships. We need to ensure that these social aspects
enhance all areas of our lives.*

EMPLOYING NEW STRATEGIES: COMPLEMENTARY HOLISTIC THERAPIES

When we decide to change our lifestyles and get serious about weight control we usually follow three routines:

1. We eat well-rounded, whole foods with minimal fat and sugar.

2. We begin a program of regular aerobic exercise and stretching.

3. We begin and follow a program of stress management.

Health care providers with a holistic orientation will probably want to add some complementary therapies to this winning trio. Perhaps you will want to add guided imagery, touch, prayer and meditation, or music. These are but a few of the alternative therapies that, when used in conjunction with a program of healing nutrition, can empower our bodies, minds, and spirits.

SUMMARY

American's have grown taller and broader. Over half of the population is now categorized as obese. The effects of fast foods and too much to do have resulted in the intake of too many comfort calories. To counteract the effects of our collective weight gain, many have turned to one or more of proliferating fad diets.

Dieting by itself is never a long-term answer to weight or health maintenance. To be effective, dieting must be accomplished by lifestyle changes that include exercise and stress management. Permanent weight loss involves breaking old habits and substituting new behaviors. Some of those new behaviors include willpower, visualization, keeping a food diary, reevaluating serving sizes, and relearning and following portion control. When we become serious about weight loss, we must assess our whole being and, when we are truly ready, embark on a holistic lifestyle change program of whole body healing.

In summary, healing with nutrition is a journey that involves building, maintaining, and maximizing your precious body, mind, and spirit with nourishing food. Now armed with new facts and insights, use these tools to have fun while adding the superior fuels of healthy foods to your life plan. Imagine yourself looking and feeling your best, and then choose one or more areas you have read about here to more fully investigate and integrate into your life plan to achieve your most desirable, healthy self.

REFERENCES

Anderson, J. W., Konz, E. C., & Jenkins, D. J. (2000). Health advantages and disadvantages of weight-reducing diets: A computer analysis and critical review. *Journal of the American College of Nutrition, 19*(5), 578–590.

Holtmeier, K. B., & Seim, H. C. (2000). The diet prescription for obesity. What works? *Minnesota Medicine, 83*(11), 28–32.

Mokdad, A. H., Serdula, M. K. , Dietz, W. H., Bowman, B. A., Marks, J. S., & Koplan, J. P. (2000). The continuing epidemic of obesity in the United States. *JAMA, 284*(13), 1650–1651.

Moloney, M.(2000). Dietary treatments of obesity. *Proceedings of the Nutrition Society, 59*(4), 601–608.

Rogers, P. J., & Smit, H. J. (2000) Food craving and food "addiction": A critical review of the evidence from a biopsychosocial perspective. *Pharmacology and Biochemical Behavior, 66*(1), 3–14

Thompson, D., Edelsberg, J., Colditz, G. A., Bird, A. P., & Oster, G. (1999). Lifetime health and economic consequences of obesity. *Archives of Internal Medicine, 159*(18), 2177–2183.

Vgontzas, A. N., Bixler, E. O., Papanicolaou, D. A., & Chrousos, G. P. (2000). Chronic systemic inflammation in overweight and obese adults. *JAMA, 283*(17), 2235; discussion 2236.

Weber, M. A., Neutel, J. M., & Smith, D. H. (2001). Contrasting clinical properties and exercise responses in obese and lean hypertensive patients. *Journal of the American College of Cardiologists, 37*(1), 169–174.

World Health Organization. (1997, June 12). Obesity epidemic puts millions at risk from related diseases. Press release. Available: http://www.who.ch.

INDEX

Date Due

BRODART, CO.   Cat. No. 23-233-003   Printed in U.S.A.